W0232386

Red Flags and Blue Lights

SECOND EDITION

Red Flags and Blue Lights

Managing Serious Spinal Pathology

Sue Greenhalgh PhD MA GD Phys FCSP
Consultant Physiotherapist, Bolton NHS
Foundation Trust, Bolton, UK

Clinical Fellow, Manchester Metropolitan University,
Manchester, UK

James Selfe DSc PhD MA GD Phys FCSP
Professor of Physiotherapy, Manchester
Metropolitan University, Manchester, UK

Foreword by
Laura Finucane and Chris Mercer

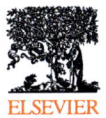

ELSEVIER

Edinburgh   London   New York   Oxford   Philadelphia   St Louis   Sydney   2019

© **2019, Elsevier Limited. All rights reserved.**
First edition 2006
Second edition 2019

The right of Sue Greenhalgh and James Selfe to be identified as authors of this work has been asserted by them in accordance with the Copyright, Designs and Patents Act 1988.

Artwork by Ruth Eaves, Medical Artist, Bolton NHS Foundation Trust © 2019. All rights reserved. Illustration not to be reproduced in whole or in part without permission of the copyright owner.

No part of this publication may be reproduced or transmitted in any form or by any means, electronic or mechanical, including photocopying, recording, or any information storage and retrieval system, without permission in writing from the publisher. Details on how to seek permission, further information about the Publisher's permissions policies and our arrangements with organizations such as the Copyright Clearance Center and the Copyright Licensing Agency, can be found at our website: www.elsevier.com/permissions.

This book and the individual contributions contained in it are protected under copyright by the Publisher (other than as may be noted herein).

Notices

Practitioners and researchers must always rely on their own experience and knowledge in evaluating and using any information, methods, compounds or experiments described herein. Because of rapid advances in the medical sciences, in particular, independent verification of diagnoses and drug dosages should be made. To the fullest extent of the law, no responsibility is assumed by Elsevier, authors, editors or contributors for any injury and/or damage to persons or property as a matter of products liability, negligence or otherwise, or from any use or operation of any methods, products, instructions, or ideas contained in the material herein.

ISBN: 978-0-7020-5510-2
Content Strategist: Poppy Garraway Smith/Serena Castelnovo
Content Development Specialist: Veronika Watkins/Carole McMurray
Project Manager: Louisa Talbott
Design: Maggie Reid
Illustration Manager: Narayanan Ramakrishnan
Illustrator: Ruth Eaves, Medical Artist, Bolton NHS Foundation Trust
Marketing Manager: Merin Thomas

Printed in China

Last digit is the print number: 9 8 7 6 5 4 3 2 1

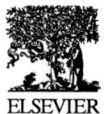

ELSEVIER

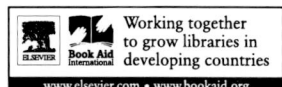

Working together
to grow libraries in
developing countries

www.elsevier.com • www.bookaid.org

Contents

Foreword

What a privilege to have been asked to write the foreword for the latest work from Sue Greenhalgh and James Selfe, *Red Flags and Blue Lights*. We have both been inspired by Sue and James's work on serious pathology in the spine, which has led the way in moving the physiotherapy profession forward in this area. In your career you may be fortunate to have the opportunity to see leaders and innovators at work; Sue and James certainly fit the bill and it has been a real honour to work closely with two such dedicated professionals. We are all standing on the shoulders of giants, and Sue and James continue to build on the work of Grieve, Gifford and countless others in pushing the management of serious spinal pathology and developing the profession.

Red Flags and Blue Lights focuses on three main pathologies: Metastatic Spinal Cord Compression, Cauda Equina Syndrome and Osteoporosis. The concentration on these three important areas reflects the clinical reality of working with this patient group and serves to give support to those treating patients with these conditions. Anyone working in this field will know Sue and James's work and might reasonably ask what this text adds. It adds depth of information and real hands-on clinical nuggets to help steer a course through the diagnosis and management of these conditions, linking to the clinician's role supporting people in taking more control of their own health.

The recent UK NHS long-term plan published in 2019 proposes that clinicians support early intervention for those at risk of osteoporosis, a condition that is often overlooked as serious pathology of the spine but which can be life-changing for patients if not managed appropriately. Chapters 3 and 4 outline the seriousness of this condition and will help clinicians to significantly impact on this agenda in preventing fractures in the future. Chapters 5 and 6 build on Sue and James's previous work in the area of CES, giving clear guidance on safe and practical management of this complex and worrying syndrome. The NHS long-term plan also goes on to discuss the importance of early diagnosis of cancer to improve survival. Chapters 7 and 8 provide helpful tools to aid in the early diagnosis of malignant spinal disease and appropriate management.

Throughout the text, clinicians are reminded of the importance of great communication and Chapter 2 provides the foundation for clear communication, including excellent advice on the difficult area of breaking bad news.

This text is a superb addition to the authors' impressive work to date and will undoubtedly improve patient care. It will be a valuable addition to any clinician's library. So, settle down and take a ride with *Red Flags and Blue Lights*. There's nothing to fear on this journey, just lots of sensible advice and practical tips. Enjoy.

Laura Finucane and Chris Mercer
2019

Acknowledgements

Our thanks go out to many who have contributed to this text. We sincerely thank you all.

Special thanks to Dr Vivek Misra, Consultant Clinical Oncologist and Lena Richards, MSCC coordinator, both of the Christie NHS Foundation Trust. Their expertise has been invaluable. Thanks to Dynamic Health CCS NHS Trust for supporting the translation of the CES cards into 28 different languages and to Jayne Davies and Kormal Bhuchhada for identifying the need to do so. Thanks also to both Dynamic Health and the MACP for hosting the free access link on their website. Our thanks must also extend to our patients who consented to share their experience with us so that they could help us to help you.

CHAPTER 1

Introduction

Only a small proportion of patients will have an identifiable cause for their back pain and these causes are serious (Hartvigsen et al., 2018).

It's Friday and it's 4 pm and you are working in a spinal assessment clinic.

Your next patient is Barbara, a 62-year-old woman. She presents with an 18-month history of low back pain (LBP) and bilateral leg symptoms. Barbara has been referred to you by the local physiotherapy department. She was previously seen by a consultant neurologist 8 months earlier and a lumbar spine magnetic resonance imaging (MRI) scan was carried out. Degenerative changes only were identified with no neurological compromise. The neurologist referred Barbara on for physiotherapy. The problem with LBP and bilateral leg pain has continued to progress very slowly with a sudden deterioration over the last 2 months. Barbara now complains of increasing hip pain, bilateral leg pain and paraesthesia in both legs. She also complains of extra-segmental numbness in both legs affecting both the anterior and posterior aspects of the legs to the ankles, with pins and needles in both feet. The paraesthesia in the feet is intermittent and particularly worse in the morning. She describes a recent onset of tripping and falling and feels as if she is losing all of the feeling in both legs. She describes feeling unsteady with poor balance.

Over the last 4 weeks, Barbara describes hesitancy in relation to bladder control, with frequency of passing small amounts of urine. She can tell when she has finished passing urine and sensation when she wipes herself after toileting is normal. She describes pain first thing in the morning as a 7/10 on a numeric pain rating scale but as the day progresses, so does the pain, increasing to 10/10. She explains that in the previous 18 months she had lost 9 kg (20 lb) in weight but this unexplained weight loss has now stabilised. This weight loss equates to approximately 10% of her body weight over an 18-month period. At the time of her first attendance, Barbara needs morphine to control her symptoms. Sleep was very disturbed due to pain and she described getting stuck in positions due to pain when she tries to roll over in bed during the night.

On examination, the unsteadiness on her legs is obvious. Barbara stands with a wide-based gait but has a fairly good range of movement. Objectively, there is no neurology to find including reflexes. From a medication perspective, she is taking the following: morphine twice a day; ibuprofen three times a day; paracetamol three times a day; pregabalin three times a day.

Past medical history

Barbara has a history of cervical spinal fusion. She underwent an operation 11 years ago for a C6–7-disc protrusion with C7 root entrapment, producing left arm pain and weakness. Complete recovery was achieved postoperatively. She is a 10 per day smoker and has smoked for 40 years, drinks minimal amounts of alcohol and has no history of tuberculosis (TB) or cancer.

What are your diagnostic alternatives?

What investigations will you organise and importantly when?

Barbara is a real case with no change to the clinical picture other than her name. Barbara's case highlights the conundrums that complex spinal conditions can bring to front-line practitioners on a daily basis. We will hear more about Barbara later in the book.

Our introduction takes us through a journey relating to back pain and serious pathology of the spine. This journey outlines both current and future challenges we, as physiotherapists, are likely to face in the changing world we practice in with an ageing population within front-line autonomous roles.

Introduction

LBP is a common and internationally significant problem which affects both men and women. In 2016, LBP was the leading cause of years lived with disability (YLDs) globally, contributing to a staggering 57.6 million YLDs in 195 countries (1990–2016). For men, LBP resulted in the highest age-standardised rates of YLDs in 133 of 195 countries, including every country in the high-income regions, central and eastern Europe, central Asia, Andean and tropical Latin America, and eastern and central sub-Saharan Africa, and most countries in Southeast Asia, North Africa and the Middle East, and western sub-Saharan Africa. For women, LBP resulted in the highest age-standardised YLD rates in 104 of 195 countries. It was the main cause of YLDs in almost all high-income, central Europe, eastern Europe, North Africa and the Middle East, and Andean and tropical Latin American countries (GBD 2016 Disease and Injury Incidence and Prevalence Collaborators, 2017). People with physically demanding jobs, physical and mental comorbities, smokers and obese individuals are more at risk of experiencing back pain (Hartvigsen et al., 2018). For most people it is not possible to identify a specific nociceptive cause for their back pain. There is only a small population who have a well-understood pathological cause, for example, fracture, cancer or infection (Hartvigsen et al., 2018). Fortunately, serious spinal pathology is usually considered as being rare, and is often estimated as just 1% of the total back pain population (CSAG, 1994). More recently, Henschke et al. (2009) reported on 1172 new presentations to primary care of acute LBP of less than 2 weeks' duration in Australia; only 0.9% were found to have a specific serious cause for their problems. Assessing for serious spinal pathology has often been likened to looking for a 'needle in a haystack'. The evidence cited above tells us, however, that the 'haystack' is actually very large and therefore we are likely to find quite a few 'needles' of varying kinds! Physiotherapists at the front end of healthcare can make a huge contribution to identifying these cases early and optimising the ultimate outcome for patients with serious spinal pathology. Eighty percent of people with acute LBP have at least one Red Flag despite less than 1% having a serious disorder (Hartvigsen et al., 2018). It is important to remember there are 163 individual items that could be considered as Red Flags: 119 items in the patient history and 44 items in the physical examination (Chartered Society of Physiotherapy (CSP), 2007). Individual Red Flags in isolation are therefore not particularly helpful. Combinations of Red Flags are far more useful in informing the clinical reasoning process and will develop over time, reinforcing the value of the 'watchful wait' approach to management of back pain.

One of the challenges in writing a new Red Flags book is deciding on what to include and what to omit as there have been many developments in this field compared to when we began our first book over a decade ago. This book pays particular attention to two specific emergency conditions which require immediate action and one pathology that requires action many years before. Currently, there is still no international consensus on which Red Flags might be useful in the identification of serious spinal pathology or on how they should be used in the clinical setting (Verhagen et al., 2016). The need for further research to provide data on the diagnostic accuracy of Red Flags was identified in 2016 after a consultation of the member organizations of the International Federation of Orthopaedic Manipulative Physical Therapists (IFOMPT), a sub group of the World Confederation for Physical Therapy (WCPT). Listed below are the four key serious pathologies which were identified as areas in which more research is urgently required:

1. vertebral fracture
2. spinal malignancy
3. spinal infection
4. cauda equina syndrome (CES)

Premkumar et al. (2018) confirm the importance of these four conditions in their review of 9940 patients attending a specialist spinal surgery centre in the USA. They reported the most common serious pathology was fracture (n=554, 5.6%), followed by tumour (n=159, 1.6%) and infection (n=120, 1.2%), with CES being the least common (n=36, 0.4%). This book therefore aims to help practitioners identify and appropriately manage (keep or refer) the two most common emergency musculoskeletal conditions of CES and metastatic spinal cord compression (MSCC). In both of these emergency conditions it may actually be necessary for you to ring an ambulance to transport the patient immediately to the appropriate surgical/hospital service; hence the title of the book *Red Flags and Blue Lights*. It is our experience within our national and international work that these two topics receive the most clinical interest and cause the most concern. You may be surprised to see we have also included chapters on osteoporosis. This is a topic we are rarely questioned about but in our opinion should be; this is reflected in the topics to be studied by the IFOMPT subgroup. Osteoporosis has a significant impact on morbidity and mortality yet is often the 'Cinderella' serious pathology ranked lower than spinal infection or, indeed, inflammatory conditions, until a significant insufficiency fracture develops and timely treatment is required. Fragility spinal fractures are the most common serious spinal pathology that presents in primary care, one of the aims here is to encourage the development of a wider public health role in line with 'making every contact count' (see Chapter 4). The effect of much earlier prophylactic interventions will, in future, hopefully reduce the need for a Blue Light to be switched on when, for instance, a retropulsed insufficiency vertebral fracture causes CES or cord compression! Underpinning all clinical work, but especially important in managing serious spinal pathology, we have also included a chapter on communication. This chapter concludes with strategies to help break bad news to patients and their relatives or carers, a skill more commonly needed in these expanded front-line roles.

This book does not cover all the possible emergency conditions for serious causes of spinal pain including masqueraders, such as infection and abdominal aortic aneurysm (AAA), or inflammatory causes, such as ankylosing spondylitis, so we urge you to embark on further reading around these other very important conditions. In addition, this book does not cover the variety of serious conditions that could cause cord or cauda equina compression but, as described, concentrates on two emergency spinal conditions (MSCC and CES) that can present to front-line practitioners. Consider in-depth additional reading in relation to other musculoskeletal masqueraders, especially when working in roles such as first contact practitioner (FCP) and interface positions. In the UK, FCP roles take the place of a general practitioner (GP) in a primary care setting. For example, consider the patient who attends with left shoulder pain (potentially a referral of heart pain) or right shoulder pain (potentially a liver or gallstones referral of pain) where differential diagnosis is critical.

Many of the conditions not discussed in this book may also require a Blue Light approach. AAA for instance is an emergency condition which has been described as 'the forgotten Red Flag' (Box 1.1). Although AAA is not discussed, we did not wish to 'forget it' as knowledge of this condition is essential for front-line practitioners, so further reading is essential. It was listed as the 15th leading cause of mortality in the United States in 2013 in adults aged between 60 and 64, and its prevalence is likely to increase significantly in association with an ageing population (Tsuchie et al., 2013). As front-line practitioners, we need to be able to identify those who need an urgent medical review and act accordingly. AAA is an abnormal widening of the aorta of more than 3 cm in diameter. It can be asymptomatic and can be fatal if diagnosed late. The majority are related to atherosclerotic changes, with 10% related to an inflammatory process of the blood vessel wall. LBP is one of the symptoms of AAA, with a high prevalence of chronic LBP amongst AAA patients (Tsuchie et al., 2013). In the UK, screening is available for men aged 65 and over using an ultrasound scan. There

BOX 1.1 Abdominal aortic aneurysm (AAA) (NHS Choices, 2017).

Symptoms
- Pulsing sensation in the abdomen
- Abdominal and or back pain that does not go away
- Can cause sudden severe abdominal and back pain if ruptures
- Dizziness
- Sweating and pallor
- Rapid heartbeat and shortness of breath
- Fainting or passing out

Those at risk
- Men aged >65 years
- Smokers past and present (×15 more likely)
- High blood pressure (×2 more likely)
- Family history in first degree relative (×4 more likely)
- Caucasian race

Reduce risks of AAA
- Stop smoking
- Healthy eating
- Exercise regularly
- Maintain healthy weight
- Reduce alcohol intake

are 6000 deaths a year in England and Wales from ruptured AAA. If a patient presents with suspected dissecting AAA, timing is critical (NHS Choices, 2017).

As stated earlier, LBP is the leading cause of YLDs globally. Managing this epidemic adds significant strain to healthcare resources. The increasing global financial and demographic challenges to healthcare have been met in many countries by efforts to change whole systems to modernise health services. In some countries, this has included a specific focus on reconsidering the roles of non-medical members of the healthcare team. There is an increasing drive towards the development of a more flexible health workforce, where different professionals are able to take on each other's traditional tasks. For example, in the UK, the National Health Service (NHS) has seen the creation of a host of new roles, including extended scope practitioners (McPherson et al., 2006) and FCPs (Salmon et al., 2017). It is clear that traditional models of physiotherapy practice are experiencing significant challenges by many of the proposed reforms that are occurring in health services internationally (Nicolls & Larmer, 2005). In 2009, Nicholls et al. expanded their debate; they describe health provision not only in New Zealand, but across the world as facing an evolving demographic profile with an ageing population, an increasing affliction of chronic disease and a reduced workforce to provide necessary healthcare (Nicholls et al., 2009). In the UK, as a result of this demographic evolution, physiotherapists are enjoying increasing autonomy and taking on new and expanded roles in a wide variety of primary care environments in both public and private sectors. As a consequence of these new roles and increased autonomy, physiotherapy practice has significantly moved 'upstream' in terms of the patient's condition; in other words, physiotherapists are now seeing many more patients at much earlier stages of their disease process, often without prior medical screening. This of course brings with it exciting new professional challenges but it also increases professional responsibility and risk, especially with respect to the timely identification and appropriate management of serious spinal pathology. For example, Levack et al. (2002) reported that in 23% of their patients, a diagnosis of metastatic spinal cord compression LBP was the first presenting symptom of malignancy. The authors highlighted that in most patients, symptoms started when they were leading normal lives in the community yet suddenly presented with an oncology emergency. Patients with serious spinal pathology will most often first present with problems to a clinician in a primary care setting within 3 weeks of the symptoms developing (Levack et al., 2002). It is therefore imperative that primary care clinicians, whether employed in the public or private sector, are prepared for this scenario and ask the relevant questions to inform appropriate keep/refer decisions and, where indicated, initiate appropriate further investigations (Fig. 1.1).

A rapidly ageing population

People worldwide are living longer; for the first time in history most people in the world can expect to live into their sixties and beyond (World Health Organization (WHO), 2015). There are currently 15.3 million people in the UK aged 60 and above; this is expected to pass the 20 million mark by 2030 and by 2040, nearly one in four people in the UK will be aged 65 or over. Similar increases in numbers are expected in the older age groups; there are currently 1.6 million people aged 85 or over and this is predicted to more than double in the next 23 years to over 3.4 million. Nearly one in five people currently in the UK will live to see their 100th birthday (Age UK, 2018). Unfortunately, despite technical advances in medicine and improvements in public health and sanitation services, older people today are not necessarily experiencing better health in their later years compared with their parents. The rising numbers of elderly are likely to put global health and social care systems under great strain. One of the most significant factors is that the pace of population ageing is much faster than in the past and, as a consequence, all countries face similar challenges to ensure

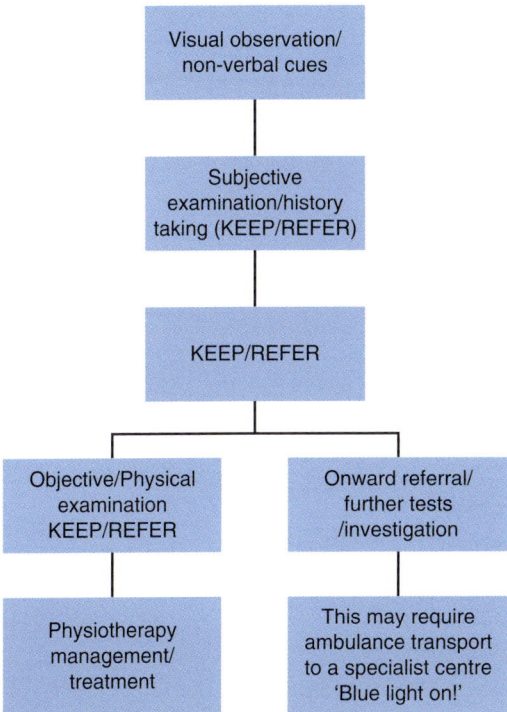

Fig. 1.1 Keep or refer at initial assessment? (Adapted from Boissonault and Umphred, 2013).

that their health and social care systems are prepared to cope with this unprecedented and rapid demographic shift (WHO, 2015). Health changes associated with age-ing are neither linear nor consistent, and they are only loosely associated with a person's age in years. Whereas some 70-year-olds enjoy extremely good health and functioning, others are frail and require significant help from others. As people age, they are more likely to experience several health conditions simultaneously. These complex health states are commonly referred to as geriatric syndromes and are often the consequence of multiple underlying factors. An holistic understanding of elderly patients is therefore required as ageing is not only potentially associated with complex health states, but is also associated with other major life transitions such as retirement, relocation from the family home to more appropriate housing and the death of friends and partners (WHO, 2015). Physical activity is really important as people get older as it can have a positive effect on health and lifestyle. For example, physical activity reduces the chance of:

- type II diabetes by 40%
- cardiovascular disease by 35%
- falls, depression and dementia by 30%
- joint and back pain by 25%
- cancers (colon and breast) by 20%

(UK Chief Medical Officers' Guidelines, 2011)

Ageing and cancer

Cancer is primarily a disease of older people, with incidence rates increasing with age for most cancers. More than a third (36% in the UK in 2013–2015) of cancers are diagnosed in people aged 75 and over (Cancer Research UK, 2015).

There are more than 200 different types of cancer, but four of them account for over half (53%) of all new cases in the UK (Cancer Research UK, 2015):

- breast
- lung
- prostate
- bowel

In some specific cancers, there is a very clear link between increasing age and the occurrence of the condition, for example, lung cancer and myeloma. There is a marked increase in the number of cases between the ages 40–49 and 50–59, and another even more dramatic increase between ages 50–59 and 60–69. Breast and prostate cancer both occur more frequently in the over 65-year-old age group. Seventy percent of all actual deaths from cancer occur in people over 65 years of age.

Ageing and osteoporosis

Osteoporosis is recognised internationally as a major healthcare problem. It is a progressive decrease in bone density particularly occurring after the age of 50; over 80% of all fractures in women over 50 are caused by osteoporosis (Osteoporosis Canada, 2018). Fractures from osteoporosis are more common than heart attack, stroke and breast cancer combined (Osteoporosis Canada, 2018). At least 1 in 3 women and 1 in 5 men will suffer from an osteoporotic fracture during their lifetime (Osteoporosis Canada, 2018). Hip and vertebral fractures are associated with reduced survival and considerable morbidity. In the European Union, there were an estimated 23.7 million vertebral fractures in 2000 and, as the population ages, it is predicted that this will rise to 37.3 million in 2050 (European Commission, 2004). However, it is important to note that despite 40,000 vertebral fractures occurring in postmenopausal British women each year, only one-third will develop clinical features (National Osteoporosis Society, 1993). Although synonymous with women, it should be remembered that, due to the increasing number of elderly people, there is also now an increased prevalence in men.

Ageing summary

The morbidity and mortality statistics presented in the previous two sections are really important to consider in light of the demographics data on the ageing population: as previously stated nearly one in four people in the UK will be aged 65 or over by 2040; therefore serious spinal pathology will be more prevalent. Let us consider this in the context of the changing nature of physiotherapy, where practice has moved 'upstream' in terms of the patient's condition, i.e. physiotherapists are now seeing patients at much earlier stages of their disease process, often without prior medical screening. Putting this together suggests that, in the future, more physiotherapists will be seeing more cancer patients, with a previously unknown cancer diagnosis, more often. They will be seeing more insufficiency vertebral fracture cases in both men and women. Therefore the identification of Red Flags is a priority when conducting diagnostic triage, especially in older patients. Although serious pathology currently occurs in what is said to be a very small percentage of patients, with a rapidly ageing population, this is likely to rise.

Changing disease profiles

Another challenge facing physiotherapy practice is the changing nature of the health of populations. For example, when we started training as physiotherapists in the early 1980s, HIV/AIDs had only recently been discovered and had not claimed any lives in the UK. TB was a condition that we learned about from a 'historical interest' perspective rather than as a condition that we were expecting to see in clinical practice; it was thought at the time that the disease would be eradicated due to the alleviation of poverty combined with the success of anti-tuberculosis drugs. After a brief period of optimism, the advent of the AIDS pandemic and the emergence of drug-resistant strains of the bacteria has resulted in TB re-emerging as a major threat to public health worldwide (WHO, 2018). TB is now a major health problem globally; it is one of the top ten causes of death worldwide and over 25% of the world's population is currently infected (WHO, 2018). Any students training today will face health conditions that we probably will never have heard of or that do not actually currently exist; for example, how many physiotherapists in the UK had heard of Ebola in 2013?

Pain experience/modulation: the challenge of identifying serious pathology in the prodromal phase

Now you feel it, now you don't!

Cancer pain is a complex phenomenon caused by a combination of inflammatory, neuropathic and ischaemic mechanisms (Falk et al., 2014). Pain arises from destruction or compression of structures such as bone, nerves or soft tissue often involving mixed nociceptor and neuropathic mechanisms. In addition, a subjective component affects the pain perceived. According to the International Association for the Study of Pain, pain is;

> *An unpleasant sensory and emotional experience associated with actual or potential tissue damage, or described in terms of such damage.*
>
> **Merskey & Bogduk, 1994.**

Hence, the resultant experience of pain is governed by cognitive and emotional stimuli, peripheral and central sensitisation, and is modified by facilitatory or inhibitory central mechanisms. Bone pain is the most common anatomical cause of pain relating to cancer. Approximately half of cancer patients complain of pain at the time of diagnosis. In addition to the compressive and/or destructive mechanisms of pain, chemicals released by the cancer cells can also mediate an inflammatory response contributing to the pain experience (Bennett, 2014). These chemical factors include:

- neural growth factors
- cytokines e.g. tumour necrosis factor (TNF)
- interleukins
- chemokines
- prostanoids
- endothelins
  (Bennett, 2014)

It is well known that in the prodromal stages (Box 1.2) of the disease process in serious spinal pathology, pain fluctuates and can even come and go, masquerading as simple mechanical back pain, militating against consistent early-disease diagnosis. We have observed this in a large number of cases presenting to us in clinical practice at an early stage in the disease process.

This fluctuation in pain is an important and sometimes very misleading observation for musculoskeletal

| **BOX 1.2** The prodromal phase.

Gould (2006) writing specifically about cancer describes three distinct clinical phases:
- Subclinical
  pathological changes but no signs and symptoms
- Prodromal
  vague, nonspecific symptoms, few if any signs
- Clinical
  well-developed signs and symptoms

physiotherapists to be aware of. Sometimes patients may not routinely consider themselves a back-pain sufferer; others consider back pain to be a common feature of daily life. Both groups of patients need to be rigorously screened for Red Flags, which should be carefully monitored over time and every time they are reviewed. The case of Rose is a good illustration of the complexities of pain in serious pathology of the spine. Rose was a 58-year-old woman who presented to an orthopaedic clinic with back pain and unknown, undiagnosed metastases of the spine. She had a 42-year history of chronic LBP. Throughout the previous decade, back pain symptoms had been episodically severe, and significantly worse over the preceding 12 months due to a lifting injury at work. Five years previously, Rose had been 'successfully' treated for breast cancer. At her first presentation, Rose presented with what appeared to be a mechanical back pain, with no leg pain, no neurological signs or symptoms and no worrying findings on objective examination. As Rose had only two Red Flags in her history (age 58 years and previous history of breast cancer), the clinician elected to observe very closely over time and treat with a gentle conservative approach. Rose quickly reported significant improvement to the therapist and was delighted with her considerable progress. She actually reported being the best she had been for 42 years! Unfortunately, the improvement was not sustained and soon after, Rose's picture deteriorated; the therapist's close observation allowed rapid investigation, onward referral and diagnosis of spinal metastases. Rose had spinal metastases, so it is puzzling as to how and why she responded so well to a conservative management approach. This is not uncommon and is something that we see time and time again; patients suffering from spinal metastases reporting improvement with gentle manual therapy, simple analgesics or even a simple exercise approach.

Nijs et al. (2015) describe one possible mechanism of pain modulation, 'brain-orchestration', which may help to explain why patients in the early stages of serious pathology often report improvement in response to physiotherapy. Stimulation of nociceptors results in action potentials transported along two primary sensory nerve types: A delta and C fibres. A delta fibres are myelinated, have a fast conduction speed and result in sharp and localised pain. C fibres, on the other hand, are unmyelinated, have a slow conduction speed and result in dull, wide spread, poorly demarcated pain. This sensory information is transmitted along these primary sensory nerve fibres to the central nervous system in the dorsal horn of the spinal cord where the nerve fibres synapse with secondary sensory nerve fibres, which can send impulses of pain to the brain. However, these synapses are controlled and modulated by local and descending neurones. Brain-orchestration can be highly effective; it can reduce the number of or even stop pain signals reaching the brain at all, so no pain is perceived. Even if the synapse is not modulated and the secondary sensory nerve fibres do transmit information to the brain, the action potential is only registered as pain if the brain perceives the signal as a threat and registers it as such, resulting in a pain experience. This dampening down of pain signals lies at the opposite end of the pain spectrum to chronic pain sufferers; both situations present significant challenges for musculoskeletal physiotherapists.

Physical stressors are cited by Nijs et al. (2015) as factors which result in nociception inhibition by endogenous analgesia. Exercise is a specific physical stressor, and Rose was given a simple paced walking regime and gentle core stability exercises. This could help to explain her significant improvement. Similarly, manual joint mobilisations have also been shown to activate descending nociceptor inhibition, inducing analgesia (Nijs et al., 2015). Sheila, a 57-year-old teacher, with a 4-week history of LBP, was treated with manual therapy techniques for 6 weeks. She was eventually diagnosed with spinal metastases with no previous diagnosis of cancer; Sheila was later found to have breast cancer. In the early stages of treatment, the treating therapist was reassured that Sheila had a 'straightforward' mechanical back problem as her only Red Flag was her age. Significantly, at each session of manual therapy, Sheila's pain was immediately reduced with an associated marked increased range of movement. Unfortunately, the improvements in pain and range of motion were short-lived and monitoring Sheila closely over time revealed emerging Red Flags. Reviewing Red flags at each consultation cannot be overemphasised. Musculoskeletal physiotherapists are in a unique position to do this, contributing to the early identification of serious diseases, which often leads to a significant impact on their outcome (Patchell et al., 2005).

Within the pain matrix proposed by Melzack (1990), the amygdala has an important role in pain signal modulation and has a key role in emotions and pain-related memory. The amygdala is a deep structure situated in the medial temporal lobe of the brain which is strongly associated with the regulation of emotion (Siegel & Sapru, 2015). Of importance is that the amygdala can be influenced by positive treatment expectations and is closely aligned to the placebo effect (Nijs et al., 2015). Sheila had responded well to a manual physiotherapy approach in the past for previous episodes of back pain. Her expectation was that she would have a positive response to treatment once again. Rose was not only taking active control of her situation by exercising to modulate her pain, but she was also confident in her physiotherapist's ability. It is possible that these positive expectations may also have contributed to the reported improvements in her condition.

It is interesting to consider the mature organism model described by Gifford (2014). Within this model, Gifford describes the human central nervous system as constantly sampling its environment, then sending information received from this sampling to the nervous system and brain. The brain interrogates the incoming information and reaches a conclusion/output. One category of outputs is altered behaviour and physiology. At an evolutionary level, could this potentially be why sleep and appetite are disturbed when serious pathology is established? Good sleep is described as linked to good recovery and healing; therefore patients with a serious condition should sleep more rather than less. However, when awake, the body can turn its attention to survival. Inability to lay supine, which is often described by patients with serious spinal pathology, could be an evolutionary means of preparing for flight. Margaret was a 49-year-old patient who presented to a spinal assessment clinic complaining of thoracic pain due to a road traffic collision. She had an undiagnosed primary breast cancer with resultant spinal metastasis. Margaret found that sleeping upright in a chair helped (Greenhalgh & Selfe, 2004). Similarly, good nutrition leads to growth; therefore could loss of appetite be a primitive evolutionary response to under-nourishing a growing malignant lesion? It is interesting to speculate if primitive evolutionary physiological changes underpin many of the contemporaneous reasons for sleep being significantly disturbed and appetite being reduced.

Safety netting

As previously stated, prodromal non-specific cancer symptoms in patients presenting early in the disease process into primary care settings can result in profound challenges to clinical reasoning for front-line clinicians responsible for diagnosis of LBP. With older patients, this can be compounded further by the coexistence of multiple and complex comorbidities. One benefit of the primary care system in the UK is the capability to follow patients up. This allows patients to be observed over time ('watchful waiting') (Cook et al., 2017), and investigations to be carried out if the symptomatology progression causes concern. One of the diagnostic tools employed during this observation over time is referred to as 'safety netting'. This is a consultation technique utilised to facilitate timely review of a patient's condition, should the need arise (Bankhead et al., 2011).

Safety netting was introduced in the seminal work of Roger Neighbour (2004) who considered this as a key feature of a good general practice consultation. Neighbour considers no patient to be safe unless the consultation includes safety netting (Neighbour, 2004). The core elements of safety netting are listed by Bankhead et al. (2011) as:

1. communicating the existence of uncertainty
2. outlining what new/changing clinical features to look out for after the consultation
3. how and where exactly to seek further help
4. what to expect about the time course of the condition; for example, when an improvement in symptoms is likely to occur and when it is expected that symptoms will have resolved completely

It is estimated that there are 300,000 new cases of cancer each year in the UK with one in three people now developing cancer at some point in their life. With an ageing population, these figures are set to rise. Bankhead et al. (2011) identify specific additional components of safety netting for GPs to implement in relation to cancer diagnosis in a primary care setting:

1. ensure specific actions are communicated to patient
2. list actions that GPs should take during or shortly after the consultation
3. organisational procedures that should be implemented at practice level

We can learn much from the hurdles that GPs face in terms of early diagnosis of cancer. For instance, although cancer appears to be common at the population level, an individual GP is said to see only 8 or 9 new cancer cases of all types in 1 year. According to the National Cancer Registration and Analysis Service (2018), cancer survival in England is lower than the European average, which in part has been attributed to late diagnosis. This in turn may be linked to unfamiliarity with the signs and symptoms of cancer due to the relatively low contact rates individual GPs have with new cancer patients. Whitaker et al. (2015) report that according to The National Cancer Intelligence Network report approximately 23% of newly diagnosed cancer patients were diagnosed as a consequence of emergency hospital presentation. Cancer patients who are diagnosed as a result of attending an emergency department have a lower survival rate than those presenting through other routes and are more likely to be elderly (Whitaker et al., 2015). Help-seeking behaviour of potential cancer sufferers is a potentially modifiable route to improving early diagnosis. Survival rates of lung cancer patients between comparable countries is said to vary significantly and it is proposed that this is mostly due to timing of diagnosis (Mitchell et al.,

2013). Understandably, there is much interest in pathways to diagnosis and factors that influence the timing of that pathway. Lower socioeconomic status, male and older age associated with lower health literacy and lower cancer symptom knowledge are likely to lead to a delay in health-seeking behaviour. Lower health expectations and lack of social support also hamper symptom interpretation. Symptom 'familiarity' leads to serious symptoms potentially being normalised as common within the social network (Whitaker et al., 2015). Long-term smokers and those with multiple comorbidities, for example, are known to take longer than average to seek healthcare for a newly presenting symptom or symptoms (Mitchell et al., 2013). Interestingly, there are significant regional and demographic variations in cancer survival across England (National Cancer Registration and Analysis Service, 2018). It is estimated that if sociodemographic inequalities were eliminated, there would be 5600 fewer patients per year diagnosed with cancer at an advanced stage. It is therefore important, as a clinician, to have a clear understanding of the needs of the population you serve to help facilitate early diagnosis.

Whitaker et al. (2015) cites the model of Pathways to Treatment as conceptualising and identifying possible areas of delay to diagnosis. This descriptive model of events begins at the detection of a bodily change, considers how the patient processes the information and considers what is described as the patient interval, in other words the time from noticing the bodily change to considering it a reason to seek healthcare advice. The pathways to treatment model then describes a component of delay as conceptually the time from decision to seek healthcare to first appointment—all critical in the quest for early diagnosis of serious spinal pathology. This is very similar to the biopsychosocial model outlined by the WHO (2001) where people pass a 'personal' threshold where they decide to seek medical help. This threshold is modified by the environment in which they live.

Easton (2016) describes Zola's triggers, first described in 1973, where symptoms alone were identified as not necessarily sufficient to prompt health-seeking behaviour. Additional triggers have an important role to play in seeking a healthcare opinion. Easton (2016) describes the five Zola trigger categories as:

- interpersonal crisis (bereavement)
- interference with social or personal relations (caring role)
- sanctioning (direction from others)
- interference with vocational or physical activity (work/exercise)
- temporalising deadline (help if not recovered by set date)

Elements of Zola's triggers were identified in a study by Stafford et al. (2014). They considered why patients with simple mechanical back pain sought urgent care. Their findings identified that the human response to severe pain was reinforced by functional loss, doubt, the need to provide care for others and the encouragement of others to attend. Conversely, if symptoms are perceived as 'normal' within the social setting, there will be less doubt and less encouragement from others to seek help early (Whitaker et al., 2015).

Whitaker et al. (2015) also cite the Competition of Cues theory which points out the effect of external stimuli as compromising the recognition of early symptoms and the interpretation of those symptoms once recognised. This was described by CES patients (Greenhalgh et al., 2015) who, in the context of severe pain, could not recognise early CES symptoms or concentrate on clinical questions being asked. In the context of severe pain these questions had no face value:

> *'What has my bladder got to do with my back?'*
> *'I don't think his questions weren't clear, I think that it was impossible to concentrate on anything other than pain management.'*
>
> **Greenhalgh et al., 2015**

Pennebaker (1982) describes the Competition of Cues theory in more detail but essentially considers:

> *In what setting will one be most likely to notice symptoms?*

Cacioppo et al. (1986) is cited by Whitaker as saying:

> *New bodily changes may go unnoticed if the external environment is high on stimulation, whereas fluctuations in normal bodily sensation may be noticed and attended to if the external environment is lacking.*

In the context of pain, this background 'noise' is almost always present in cases of serious pathology of the spine. With the addition of poor sociodemographic features, recognition of early symptoms is even harder.

Conclusion/summary

Extracts from the CSP briefing paper Learning from Litigation: Cauda Equina Syndrome (Chartered Society of Physiotherapy, 2014) provide a very useful summary to this introductory chapter. Physiotherapists see many patients with back pain, a large number of whom may come directly to see a physiotherapist without seeing a doctor first. As autonomous and accountable diagnostic practitioners, physiotherapists of all levels of experience need to be able to identify those patients who need urgent medical review and act accordingly, in other words refer them. Physiotherapists should:

- do a thorough subjective and objective examination of the spine
- document the examination to demonstrate a clear clinical reasoning and decision-making process; well-designed examination templates for the spine are recommended
- where possible, record the actual time symptoms occurred/events happened
- record both positive and negative neurological examination findings and clearly document this
- check Red Flag questions thoroughly
- make sure to act on Red Flag findings

Those actions need to be in a timely manner

We still do not know what to do with Barbara. We have not forgotten her; keep her case presentation in mind as you read on (Fig. 1.2).

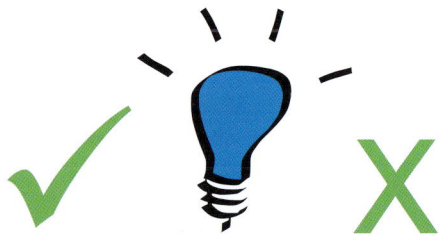

Fig. 1.2 Is the blue light on or off?

References

Age UK. Later life fact sheet. 2018. http://www.ageuk.org.uk/Documents/EN-GB/Factsheets/Later_Life_UK_factsheet.pdf?dtrk=true.

Bankhead C, Heneghan C, Hewitson P, Thompson M. *Safety Netting to Improve Early Cancer Diagnosis in Primary Care; Development of Consensus Guidelines.* Cancer Safety Netting Report, Department of Primary Care. University of Oxford; 2011.

Bennett M. Definition and pathophysiology of complex cancer pain. In: Sharma M, Simpson K, Bennett M, Gupta S, eds. *Practical Management of Complex Cancer Pain.* Oxford: Oxford University Press; 2014.

Boissonault W, Umphred D. Differential diagnosis phase 1: medical screening by the therapist. Chapter 7. In: Umphred D, Lazaro R, Roller M, Burton G, Mosby, eds. *Neurological Rehabilitation.* 6th ed. Elsevier; 2013.

Cacioppo JT, Andersen BL, Turnquist DC, Petty RE. In: Andersen BL, ed. *Psychophysiological Comparison Processes: Interpreting Cancer Symptoms Women With Cancer: Psychological Perspectives.* New York, NY, USA: Springer; 1986:142–171.

Cancer Research UK. 2015. http://www.cancerresearchuk.org/health-professional/cancer-statistics/incidence/common-cancers-compared.

Chartered Society of Physiotherapy. *Clinical Guidelines for the Effective Physiotherapy Management of Persistent Low Back Pain.* London; 2007.

Chartered Society of Physiotherapy. Learning from litigation. *Cauda Equina Syndrome.* 2014. http://www.csp.org.uk/publications/learning-litigation-cauda-equina-syndrome-ces.

Cook C, George S, Reiman M. Red flag screening for low back pain: nothing to see here, move along: a narrative review. *Br J Sports Med.* 2017;58:493–496.

CSAG. *Report of a Clinical Standards Advisory Group on Back Pain.* HMSO; 1994.

Easton G. *Great Britain: The Appointment.* Robinson; 2016.

European Commission. *Health Statistics. Key Data on Health 2002 (data 1970-2001), European Commission*; 2004.

Falk S, Bannister K, Dickinson A. Cancer Pain Physiology. *Br J Pain.* 2014;8(4):154–162.

GBD 2016 Disease and Injury Incidence and Prevalence Collaborators. Global, regional, and national incidence, prevalence, and years lived with disability for 328 diseases and injuries for 195 countries, 1990–2016: a systematic analysis for the Global Burden of Disease Study 2016. *Lancet.* 2017;390:1211–1259.

Gifford L. *The Nerve Root: Aches and Pains/Nerve Root.* CNS Press; 2014:P567.

Gould BE. *Pathophysiology for the Health Professions*. 3rd ed. Philadelphia: Saunders; 2006.

Greenhalgh S, Selfe J. Margaret: a tragic case of spinal Red Flags and Red Herrings. *Physiotherapy*. 2004;90(2):73–76.

Greenhalgh S, Truman C, Webster V, Selfe J. An investigation into the patient experience of cauda equina syndrome (CES). *Physiother Pract Res*. 2015;36:23–31.

Hartvigsen J, Hancock M, Kongsted A, et al. Low back pain 1: what low back pain is and why we need to pay attention. Lancet Low Back Pain Series Working Group. *Lancet*. 2018. https://doi.org/10.1016/s0140-6736(18)30480-X.

Henschke N, Mayer C, Refshauge K, et al. Prevalence of and screening for serious spinal pathology in patients presenting to primary care settings with acute low back pain. *Arthritis Rheum*. 2009;60:3072–3080.

Jull G, Moore A, Falla D, et al. *Grieve's Modern Musculoskeletal Physiotherapy*. 4th ed. London: Elsevier; 2015:9–11.

Levack P, Graham J, Collie D, et al. Don't wait for a sensory level–listen to the symptoms: a prospective audit of the delays in diagnosis of malignant cord compression. *Clin Oncol*. 2002;14:472–480.

McPherson K, Kersten K, George S, et al. A systematic review of evidence about extended roles for allied health professionals. *J Health Serv Res Policy*. 2006;11(4):240–247.

Melzack R. Phantom limbs and the concept of a neuromatrix. *Trends Neurosci*. 1990;13(3):88–92.

Merskey H, Bogduk N. Part III: Pain Terms, A Current List with Definitions and Notes on Usage. *Classification of Chronic Pain*. 2nd ed. Seattle: IASP Task Force on Taxonomy; 1994;209–214. https://www.iasp-pain.org/Education/Content.aspx?ItemNumber=1698.

Mitchell E, Rubin G, Maclead U. Understanding diagnosis of lung cancer in primary care: qualitative synthesis of significant audit reports. *Br J Gen Pract*. 2013;63:E37–E46.

National Cancer Registration and Analysis Service. Routes to Diagnosis. 2018. http://www.ncin.org.uk/publications/routes_to_diagnosis.

National Osteoporosis Society. *Menopause and Osteoporosis Therapy Practice Nurse Manual*. Wells: St Andrews Press; 1993.

Neighbour R. *The Inner Consultation*. 2nd ed. Oxford: Radcliffe Publishing; 2004.

NHS Choices. Abdominal Aortic Aneurysm. 2017. https://www.nhs.uk/conditions/abdominal-aortic-aneurysm.

Nicolls D, Larmer P. Possible futures for physiotherapy: an exploration of the New Zealand context. *N Z J Physiother*. 2005;33(2):55–60.

Nicholls D, Reid D, Larmer P. Crisis, what crisis? Revisiting possible futures for physiotherapy. *N Z J Physiother*. 2009;37(3):105–114.

Nijs J, De Kooning M, Beckwee D, Vaes P. The neurophysiology of pain and pain modulation: Modern pain neuroscience for musculoskeletal physiotherapists. In: *Grieve's Modern Musculoskeletal Physiotherapy 4th ed.* London: Elsevier; 2015:8-18.

Patchell RA, Tibbs PA, Regine WF. Direct decompressive surgical resection in the treatment of spinal cord compression caused by metastatic cancer: a randomised trial. *Lancet.* 2005;266:643–648.

Pennebaker JW. Perceptual processes I: competition of cues. In: *The Psychology of Physical Symptoms.* New York, NY: Springer; 1982.

Premkumar A, Godfrey W, Gottschalk M, Boden S. Red Flags for low pain are not always really red. *J Bone Joint Surg Am.* 2018;100: 368–374.

Salmon P, Humphreys K, Price J, Smith C, Heaton R. Can physiotherapy first contact practitioners reduce the burden on general practitioners and improve the management of musculoskeletal conditions? *Physiother Suppl.* 2017;103(1):143.

Siegel A, Sapru H. *Essential Neuroscience.* 3rd ed. Lippincott Williams & Wilkins Baltimore; 2015.

Stafford V, Greenhalgh S, Davidson I. Why do patients with simple mechanical back pain seek urgent care. *Physiother.* 2014;100(1):66–72.

Tsuchie H, Miyakoshi N, Kasukawa Y, et al. High prevalence of abdominal aortic aneurysm in patients with chronic low back pain. *Tohoku J Exp Med.* 2013;230(2):83–86.

UK Chief Medical Officers' Guidelines. 2011. Start Active, Stay Active. https://www.gov.uk/government/uploads/system/uploads/attachment_data/file/541233/Physical_activity_infographic.PDF.

Verhagen AP, Downie A, Popal N, Maher C, Koes BW. Red Flags presented in current low back pain guidelines: a review. *Eur Spine J.* 2016;25:2788–2802. https://doi.org/10.1007/s00586-016-4684-0.

Whitaker K, Scott S, Wardle J. Applying symptom appraisal models to understand socio demographic differences in response to cancer symptoms; a research agenda. *Br J Cancer.* 2015;112(suppl 1):S27–S34.

WHO. *International Classification of Functioning, Disability and Health.* Geneva: WHO; 2001.

WHO. Ageing and Health Fact Sheet N°404 September 2015. http://www.who.int/mediacentre/factsheets/fs404/en/.

WHO. Tuberculosis infection and transmission. 2018. http://www.who.int/mediacentre/factsheets/fs104/en/.

CHAPTER 2

Communication

There is something unnerving about hearing bad news about someone's health before they do. It's uninvited intelligence and brings a guilty burden.

In the next 10 minutes my task is to lob a hefty black rock into the still, bright water of Mr DG's world.

(Easton, 2016)

Diagnostic process

The diagnostic process requires an in-depth subjective history at each consultation along with a detailed assessment of the neurological and activity status. A patient is said to seek help from a front-line practitioner within 3 weeks of the symptoms of cancer-related serious pathology appearing (Levack et al., 2002).The subjective history is the most important aspect of the examination process, especially when attempting to identify early serious spinal pathology. In line with the principles of 'watchful waiting', reviewing Red Flags at each consultation is essential as disease processes can change over time.

Subjective examination

Early in the disease process, this is the most important aspect of the consultation. It is only later in the disease process that the objective examination reveals significant findings. The difficulty with diagnosing serious spinal conditions early and the catastrophic outcomes of delayed diagnosis are widely documented (Levack et al., 2002). Good communication skills are vital to allow us to gain an understanding of the patient's world by achieving an understanding of what the patient's symptoms are. The important items to screen within the subjective history are Red Flags. It is well recognised that the presence of Red and Yellow Flags are not mutually exclusive (Greenhalgh & Selfe, 2017). The clinical reasoning process essentially combines a biopsychosocial assessment alongside Red Flag screening to get a full picture of the current clinical presentation. Establishing the history of the present condition in detail is essential as timing is of paramount importance.

At this point it is worth reflecting on the definition of communication according to the dictionary:

Imparting or interchange of thoughts, opinions, or information by speech, writing, or signs.

(Dictionary.com, 2018)

This particular definition is relatively narrow when we consider the complexity of a subjective examination conducted with a patient in severe pain whom we have never previously met. In the UK, the Health and Care Professions Council (HCPC) (an independent regulatory body responsible for setting and maintaining standards of conduct, performance and ethics (SCPE)) lists communication as a standard of practice (standard 2) Health Care Professions Council (HCPC), 2016.

Specifically, they list the following key communication skills:

- You must listen to service users and carers and take account of their needs and wishes

- You must give service users and carers the information they want or need, in a way they can understand
- You must make sure that, where possible, arrangements are made to meet service users' and carers' language and communication

Therefore not only is good communication a core skill in physiotherapy practice, it is also a regulatory requirement which can have grave repercussions if breached. In the clinical context, communication skills are honed over time with the experience of many hours of patient contact (patient mileage). However, what is sometimes overlooked is that patients need to understand the relevance of the questions physiotherapists ask as they may not fully appreciate the importance of the question or of the subsequent consequences in relation to the answers they give, especially in the context of severe pain (Greenhalgh et al., 2015). One of the key problems in communication is the technical medical language used by clinicians (addressed by the second bullet point above).

We often think of strong communication skills in the clinical setting as consisting of good use of patient language in our spoken word along with good listening skills, and empathic use of body language such as eye contact, nodding, facial expressions, etc.

Langridge et al. (2015) go further and suggest:

> The emotional component that interlinks with the cognitive element of the clinical examination is generated by the clinicians' empathy and the ability to interpret and appreciate the patient experience enhancing the patients' sense of being listened to and understood.

The use of communication in the clinical reasoning process consists of even more, some aspects that we understand and others yet to be identified and defined properly. It is interesting to consider a study by Donker et al. (2016), who carried out a prospective cohort study of patients in 44 general practices across the Netherlands and considered the cancer-related gut feeling of the GPs. The predictive value for cancer relating to gut feeling was 35%, which increased not only with the patients' but also with the GPs' age, highlighting the importance of experience.

What is gut feeling?

Donker et al. (2016) cite Stolper (2011) as suggesting the following:

> *The gut feeling emerges as a consequence of non-analytical processing of available information and knowledge.*

Donker et al. (2016) suggests that a gut feeling gives a sense of alarm and define it as:

> *...an uneasy feeling perceived by a general practitioner as he or she is concerned about a possible adverse outcome, even though the specific indications are lacking.*

Easton (2016) confirms that, during initial medical appointments, diagnostic formulas are important but these are used and interpreted alongside other, more subtle clues:

> *I've heard it said that doctors often make their diagnoses within the first thirty seconds of seeing a patient or hearing about their symptoms.*

These gut feelings and tuning into very subtle issues in patients' presentation are very important and are often the norm when working at an advanced level in this area of serious spinal pathology. This is especially important when service specifications present time pressures for the consultation. However, equally important is picking up on more overt but non-verbal clues before the patient even speaks. For example, when Edward was called in from the waiting room for his appointment, both he and his partner looked extremely anxious. He stood with the aid of his partner with great difficulty. He walked towards the clinician with a wide-based, high-tone antalgic gait while leaning heavily on his partner. This clearly was not a result of the simple L5/S1 disc bulge reported in the referral letter. Edward was in fact diagnosed with a T10/11 central disc bulge with *ligamentum flavum* hypertrophy and calcification causing significant cord compression. Edward underwent emergency surgery and made a complete recovery.

In a previous paper, we also described John, who was a 64-year-old male (Greenhalgh & Selfe, 2003):

> …leaning heavily on the reception desk obviously in a great deal of discomfort when first seen. He was trying hard to smile despite his obvious discomfort. He appeared unwell with a sallow complexion, slightly dishevelled appearance and poorly fitting clothes. He moved to a chair in reception and sat down and soon began to half lie onto the next chair. Within 2 minutes he stood up and leant against a cupboard. Clearly his behaviour demonstrated excruciating pain. He came into the treatment room but by this stage it was already apparent that something serious was wrong.

John was diagnosed with a malignant myeloma of T12, and underwent a vertebrectomy. He survived and 12 months later was living a relatively normal life at home.

In their study of GPs, Donker et al., (2016) confirm that few Red Flags, if any, exist early in the disease process of serious pathology of the spine. It was not only knowledge of Red Flags that was found to be important but GP and patient characteristics were also cited as significant. These findings confirm an earlier systematic review (Henschke et al., 2013) that evaluated 22 clinical features used to screen patients with low back pain for malignancy. This found only four clinical features which, when used in isolation, were useful to raise the probability of malignancy:

- a previous history of cancer, positive likelihood ratio (LR+)=23.7
- elevated erythrocyte sedimentation rate (ESR) (LR+=18.0)
- reduced haematocrit (LR+=18.2)
- overall clinician judgement (LR+=12.1)

It is interesting to see 1 of these 4 items was overall clinician judgement. Together, these studies suggest much more needs to be done to investigate 'gut feeling' as a tool in the clinical reasoning process. In the absence of significant combinations of Red Flags, what is it that is transmitted from the patient to the clinician that triggers alarm bells early in the disease process?

Breaking bad news

Breaking bad news is included in the core curriculum of medical training but not necessarily in undergraduate physiotherapy training. Less complicated aspects of breaking bad news sensitively will fit within the routine scope of physiotherapy practice and require little adjustment to the clinical setting. However, the more serious side of breaking bad news is more likely to sit at an advanced practice level and require careful preparation prior to the consultation. The responsibility for breaking bad news to patients may be determined by local policy as in some areas this will fall to the GP rather than to the physiotherapist. It is important to work within your scope of practice and adhere to these local frameworks.

Our communication skills are important throughout the patient pathway of care, not least when it comes to the vital skill of breaking bad news:

> *Communicating bad news to patients well is not an optional skill; it is an essential part of professional practice.*
> **(Department of Health (DOH), 2003)**

Bad news is essentially in the eye of the beholder, but numerous definitions of bad news generally suggest information which:

> *...adversely and seriously affects an individual's view of his or her future.*
> **(DOH, 2003)**

In the musculoskeletal physiotherapy domain, this bad news is on a sliding scale but usually requires complex communication skills. Bad news may include information which many experienced physiotherapists come to regard as routine, for example informing a patient that:

- despite many medical advances, there is still no simple answer to relieving chronic back pain
- following an exercise regime needs to be a lifelong activity incorporated into the patient's self-management journey
- the pain is unlikely to go away

However, even this 'routine' information needs to be carefully communicated to the sufferer as this may have a significant impact on well-being and perceptions of future choices in life. Information relating to the possibility of a life-limiting disease is much less likely to be common practice, especially in a musculoskeletal setting, and its delivery must be very carefully considered. It must not be underestimated that this information can be upsetting not only for the patient and family but also for the clinician. This is particularly true when the information being relayed regards a potentially serious diagnosis. At this end of the sliding scale, preparation needs to be meticulous.

Breaking bad news well is an essential component of expert practice. The skill of breaking bad news well involves a multifaceted combination of verbal and non-verbal communication and begins even before the patient and clinician are in the room together. In relation to potentially serious communication, a strategy for breaking bad news is suggested by a number of authorities and always begins with a stepwise approach, initially by preparing yourself, not just with the patient information and how you are going to deliver it, but also emotionally (Fig. 2.1). A GP, Graham Easton, illustrates this well in the quote from his book 'The Appointment' (Easton, 2016) at the beginning of this chapter. It is worth taking time to prepare yourself, respecting confidentiality, by discussing the situation with a colleague, talking through your proposed approach and rehearsing out loud what you are going to say. Consider what questions you may be asked and what responses you may give; invite the patient to ask questions and reassure them that no question is stupid (Moss, 2015). Good preparation can significantly strengthen how this difficult situation is approached (Fig. 2.2).

Next, consider the environment—switch off mobile phones, divert desk telephones, eliminate disturbances or at least keep them to a minimum. Prepare the room with

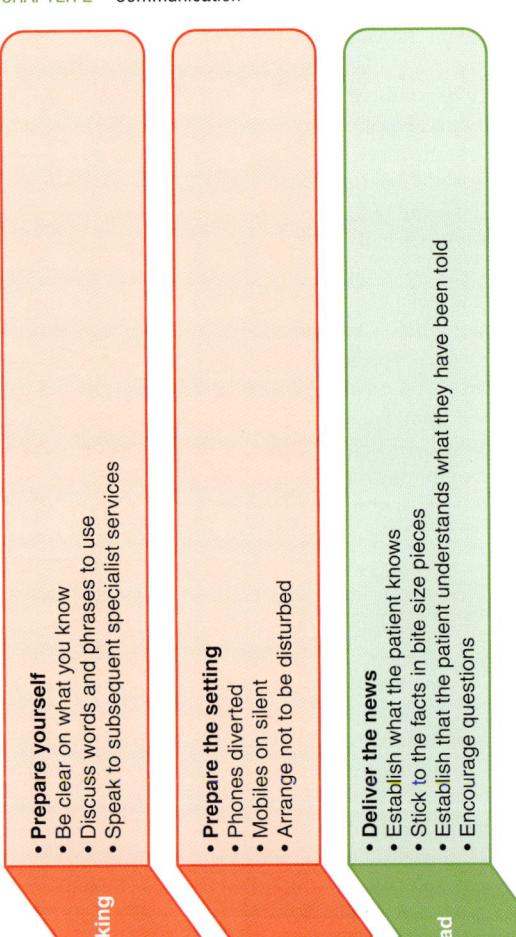

Breaking

- **Prepare yourself**
- Be clear on what you know
- Discuss words and phrases to use
- Speak to subsequent specialist services

- **Prepare the setting**
- Phones diverted
- Mobiles on silent
- Arrange not to be disturbed

Bad

- **Deliver the news**
- Establish what the patient knows
- Stick to the facts in bite size pieces
- Establish that the patient understands what they have been told
- Encourage questions

Fig. 2.1 Steps in breaking bad news.

Confirm next steps
- Ensure confirmation with specialist services first where necessary
- Encourage draft list of questions before next consultation with specialist services

Conclude consultation
- Ensure all questions answered
- Confirm next steps
- Give contact details to patient for subsequent questions if necessary

News

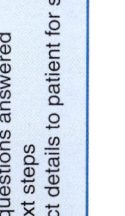

Fig. 2.1, cont'd

Patient's name/address: Hospital number:	Date and time of interview:
Location:	Names of those present:
Name: Position/relationship:	Clinical diagnosis:
Clinical options for future management and immediate plan discussed:	Detail of the words used when breaking the bad news: 'What do you think may be the cause of your problem?' 'I'm afraid that I have some bad news' 'Your investigation shows...'

Fig. 2.2 Template to record breaking bad news.

Copy to general practitioner:	Onward referral:
Referral to palliative care team: yes/no	
Filled in patient's notes along with referral to others	Signature of the clinician:
	Date:

Fig. 2.2, cont'd

no barriers between the patient and the clinician if possible; it may be worth having tissues and a glass of water to hand (DOH, 2003). Ideally, have someone to accompany you, the clinician, and someone to accompany the patient, although this is often not possible. There could potentially be four people in the clinical room at the time of the consultation. There may also be an interpreter present. If this is the case, the interpreter will also need to be prepared for the information that they are about to convey.

Deliver the sensitive information in bite size pieces avoiding jargon and do not underestimate the skill of saying nothing if there is an outburst of emotion. Easton (2016) describes giving this type of information following a 'chunk and check' approach. Be empathic and allow sufficient time for the information to be assimilated or for the emotional reaction to stabilise. This can make all the difference (Moss, 2015). Brewin (1996) makes an important point by citing Richard Asher as arguing that the art of communication is knowing:

> ...when to probe and when to leave alone, when to chide and when to reassure, when to speak and when to keep silent.

Easton (2016) describes an aide memoir to facilitate this type of consultation—the SPIKES model of breaking bad news:

- **S:** setting up the interview
- **P:** assess the **P**atient's perception
- **I:** obtain the patient's **I**nvitation to know more
- **K:** give **K**nowledge and information to the patient, keeping it simple
- **E:** address patient's **E**motions with empathy
- **S:** have a **S**trategy and summarise

Prepare the patient for bad news and gain an understanding of their perceptions of the current situation. For example, Easton (2016) suggests phrases such as

I'm afraid the test results are not what we had hoped for.

This will help to prepare the patient for what is to come next. As a physiotherapist, ensure you remain within your scope of practice and stick to what you know are the facts. For example:

I am sorry to tell you that your investigation shows…

From here more tests will be needed to investigate this further.

As opposed to

I am sorry to tell you that you have spinal metastases.

The latter could be incorrect if the investigations are based on a magnetic resonance imaging (MRI) scan alone; further tests will be necessary and the definitive diagnosis confirmed by more specialist services.

As physiotherapists, delivering bad news about the presence of a potentially serious condition is likely to be prior to the ultimate diagnosis and prognosis being confirmed. It is therefore vitally important to highlight this fact by using a phrase such as

Further tests and expertise are now required.

Ensure you conclude the consultation in a compassionate way, clarifying the next steps, and give contact details for after the consultation (Moss, 2015). It is common that many questions occur to the patient after they have left the consultation and the immediate shock has begun to sink in.

Do not underestimate how you, the clinician, will feel emotionally; drained and exhausted are not uncommon feelings.

> *His parting words were 'Thank you, you are the only one who has listened and you seem to know what's wrong, I'll see you again'. The physiotherapist's (SW) immediate thought was 'I don't know what is wrong, but I'm sure it's serious and I'm not sure I will see you again!'*
>
> **(Greenhalgh & Selfe, 2003)**

Clinical supervision and peer support are essential for you to be able to reflect on your experience and unburden yourself of that emotion.

Psychological experiments have confirmed that the bearer of bad news frequently experiences strong emotions, such as anxiety and fear, at the prospect of delivering bad news (Baile et al., 2000). Baile et al. (2000) go on to argue that clinicians prepared with a strategy to approach breaking bad news can experience less anxiety and reduce their risk of burnout. Be prepared; preparation is the key no matter how experienced you are.

In addition, offer to speak to family members if the patient wishes you to do so; another communication challenge. Christina is a lady who had possible spinal metastasis evident on an MRI scan. Christina's immediate response to hearing this news was

'*How am I going to tell my 85-year-old dad? He is in the waiting room…will you tell him?*'

The clinician enters the waiting room.

'*Mr D, Christina's father, would you like to come in please…*'

References

Baile WF, Buckman R, Lenzi R, Glober G, Beale EA, Kudelka AP. SPIKES-A six-step protocol for delivering bad news: application to the patient with cancer. *Oncologist*. 2000;5(4):302–311.

Brewin T. *Relating to the Relatives; Breaking Bad News Communication and Support*. Oxford: Radcliffe Medical Press; 1996.

Department of Health, Social Services & Public Safety. *Breaking Bad News; Regional Guidelines Developed from Partnerships in Caring (2000) DHSSPS*; 2003.

Dictionary.com. (2018). http://www.dictionary.com/browse/communication.

Donker G, Wiersma E, van der Hoek L, Heins M. Determinants of general practitioner's cancer-related gut feelings–a prospective cohort study. *BMJ Open*. 2016;6:e012511.

Easton G. *The Appointment*. UK: Constable & Robinson; 2016.

Greenhalgh S, Selfe J. Malignant myeloma of the spine. *Physiotherapy*. 2003;89(8):486–488.

Greenhalgh S, Truman C, Webster V, Selfe J. An investigation into the patient experience of cauda equina syndrome (CES). *Physiother Pract Res*. 2015;36:23–31.

Greenhalgh S, Selfe J. Screen for Red Flags first: don't take the bio out of biopsychosocial. In: Porter S, ed. *Psychologically Informed Physiotherapy*. Elsevier; 2017.

Health and Care Professions Council (HCPC). Standards of conduct, performance and ethics (SCPE). http://www.hcpc-uk.org/publications/standards/index.asp?id=38; 2016.

Henschke N, Maher C, Ostelo R, de Vet H, Macaskill P, Irwig L. *Red Flags to Screen for Malignancy in Patients with Low-Back Pain (Review)*. The Cochrane Collaboration. Wiley; 2013.

Langridge N, Roberts L, Pope C. The clinical reasoning processes of extended scope physiotherapists assessing patients with low back pain. *Man Ther*. 2015;20(6):745–750.

Levack P, Graham J, Collie D, et al. Don't wait for a sensory level - listen to the symptoms: a prospective audit of the delays in diagnosis of malignant cord compression. *Clin Oncol*. 2002;14:472–480.

Moss B. *Communication Skills in Health and Social Care*. SAGE; 2015.

Stolper E, Van de Wiel M, Van Royen P, et al. Gut feelings as a third track in general practitioners' diagnostic reasoning. *J Gen Int Med*. 2011;26:197–203.

CHAPTER 3

Osteoporosis: Diagnosis

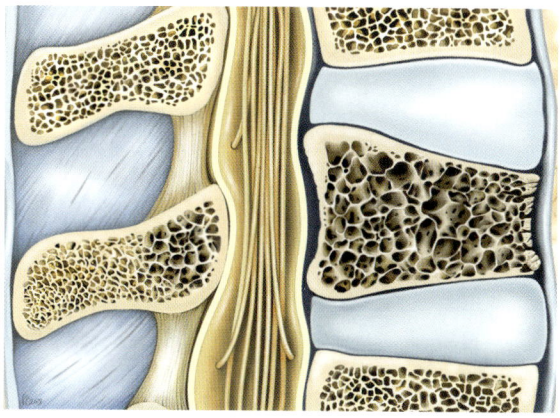

Osteoporosis.

Although osteoporosis is not traditionally considered a Blue Light medical condition where you need to call an ambulance immediately, it can progress to present as such and these numbers are likely to increase if this silent epidemic is not addressed. Every year 300,000 insufficiency fractures are sustained from a minor injury. Many could have been prevented with early diagnosis and treatment (National Osteoporosis Society, 2015). We can make a significant difference by giving the correct advice at an early stage to those at risk to prevent a serious situation from developing years later.

Marjorie was a 75-year-old woman who presented to an orthopaedic interface clinic with a sudden onset of severe low back pain. Marjorie had sustained an osteoporotic vertebral fracture of L4 and L5 that had retropulsed into the spinal canal causing reported cauda equina compression on magnetic resonance imaging (MRI). At that stage, Marjorie had no symptoms of cauda equina syndrome (CES) (see Chapter 5). Despite her age, Marjorie was surprised to learn that she was osteoporotic and did not recall having ever received any advice on bone health protection when she was younger. Although Marjorie had no symptoms of CES, she was now in a situation that could become an emergency surgical condition at any moment and for which the Blue Light would be on. Yet decades ago, as a young woman, Marjorie was at risk of osteoporosis when the Blue Light was not even on the horizon. Marjorie could have had help and advice throughout her youth and young adulthood that could have helped maximise her bone health. More needs to be done from a public health perspective to avoid cases like Marjorie presenting needlessly as an emergency decades later. Osteoporosis is often seen as an inevitable consequence of ageing (Gosch et al., 2014). However, more needs to be done to change perceptions as it could represent an exciting opportunity for physiotherapists to embrace known methods of prevention and treatment confirmed by extensive research (Bombak & Hanson, 2016).

As we alluded to in the introduction, some readers will find it surprising to see two chapters devoted to osteoporosis in a book dedicated to emergency serious spinal pathologies. However, Premkumar et al. (2018) highlight the importance of osteoporosis in their review of 9940 patients attending a specialist spinal surgery centre in the USA. They reported the most common serious pathology

Who it affects

People infographic

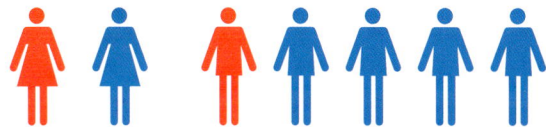

1 in 2 Women   1 in 5 Men

People over the age of 50, **who will break a bone** mainly as a result of poor bone health.

Fig. 3.1 Gender difference in osteoporotic fractures. (Reproduced courtesy of National Osteoporosis Society 2015, with permission.)

was fracture (n=554, 5.6%). Bombak & Hanson (2016) state that osteoporosis can result in fractures leading to pain, deformity, ongoing disability, reduced quality of life, loss of independence, residential care and death. In some studies minimal trauma vertebral fractures are associated with a 2–8 times increased risk of mortality (Hartvigsen et al., 2018).

Osteoporosis is the most common bone disease in humans. It affects females significantly more than males (Fig. 3.1). Osteoporosis progresses much more rapidly in women compared with men due to hormonal changes associated with the menopause. Postmenopausal loss of bone mass can be as great as 5% per year due to depletion of hormonal levels. From a clinical perspective it is important to establish when the menopause occurred. It is commonly seen that fractures start to emerge as a clinical problem 10 to 15 years post menopause.

- 1 in 2 women aged >50 will break a bone
- 1 in 5 men aged >50 will break a bone
- 1 in 5 women who have broken a bone break 3 or more before diagnosis

(National Osteoporosis Society, 2015)

The skeleton contains the vast majority of the body's calcium stores. The bony skeleton has five main functions:

- structural
- provides mobility (muscle attachment sites)
- support and protection of vital organs (heart and lungs)
- store for essential minerals
- blood cell production

When the dietary supply of calcium is inadequate, bone tissue is quickly resorbed from the skeleton. Optimal levels of calcium in the circulatory system are vital in maintaining vascular contraction and vasodilatation, muscle function, nerve transmission, intracellular signalling and hormonal secretion (Ross et al., 2011). Classic pain behaviours and coping strategies such as lack of exercise, obesity, smoking and excessive use of alcohol can not only contribute to cancer risk, but also risk of osteoporosis (Greenhalgh & Selfe, 2017).

The National Osteoporosis Foundation points out that there is a critical need for more research concentrating on bone health in youth (Weaver et al., 2016). During childhood, bones grow and repair very quickly, but this process slows with age. Bone length ceases to increase between the ages of 16 and 18, but bones continue to increase in density until the late 20s. Bone density is said to begin to reduce from approximately 35 years of age (Harding, 2017). Women lose bone rapidly in the first few years after menopause due to falling levels of oestrogen. Osteoporosis is defined as low bone mineral density (BMD) and is often associated with low-impact fractures. The most common fracture sites are:

- spine
- wrist
- hip
- pelvis

(Gosch et al., 2014)

Osteoporosis is known as the silent epidemic and affects millions of people worldwide. As stated earlier, osteoporosis was once thought to be an inevitable consequence of older age. However, advancements in non-invasive diagnostics and pharmaceutical interventions have revolutionised the management of osteoporosis and so the idea that it is an inevitable part of the ageing process has been dispelled (Cooper & Harvey, 2012). Despite its prevalence, awareness, diagnosis and management of osteoporosis broadly speaking remain poor and, although there have been significant advances in diagnosis and treatment over the last two decades, the impact of osteoporosis around the world remains largely unchanged. Postmenopausal osteoporosis expenses are expected to double by the year 2050 (Gosch et al., 2014). Short reproductive cycle as a result of late menarche and early menopause is directly related to low BMD (Ito et al., 1995).

The development of osteoporosis is associated with a variety of risk factors (Box 3.1) (National Institute of Arthritis and Musculoskeletal and Skin Diseases, 2016; National Osteoporosis Foundation, 2017).

Vitamin D is essential in the process of absorbing ingested calcium from the digestive system into the blood stream. Low levels of vitamin D (Box 3.2) are therefore a major risk factor for the development of osteoporosis.

BOX 3.1 Risk factors for the development of osteoporosis.

- Female
- Over 50 years
- Low body weight/being small and thin
- Broken bones or height loss
- Smoking (can lead to lower bone density and higher risk of fracture)
- A high intake of alcohol (>4 units of alcohol per day can double the risk of hip fracture). The risk of vertebral and hip fractures in men increases greatly with heavy alcohol intake, particularly with long-term intake
- Amenorrhea (menstruation is often suppressed by medication in young women with learning disabilities)
- Early menopause (i.e. aged below 45 years)
- Inflammatory conditions e.g. rheumatoid arthritis, Crohn's disease and chronic obstructive pulmonary disease (COPD)
- Conditions that affect the hormone-producing glands, e.g. an overactive thyroid gland (hyperthyroidism) or an overactive parathyroid gland (hyperparathyroidism)
- Family history of osteoporosis, particularly history of a hip fracture in a parent before the age of 75 years
- Long-term use of medications that affect bone strength or hormone levels, such as oral prednisolone
- Poor diet lacking in calcium, vitamin D, fruit and vegetables
- Too much protein, sodium and caffeine
- Malabsorption problems
- Vitamin D deficiency
- Inactive lifestyle

As with all serious pathology of the spine conditions, some Red Flag items have a higher weighting or risk than others but combinations of factors increase risk. This principal also holds true in osteoporosis. Perhaps

BOX 3.2 Factors influencing vitamin D levels (Hagen, 2011).

Sunlight

The amount of exposure to sunlight needed to maintain healthy bone mineral density depends on a number of variables

- Latitude
- Altitude
- Time of year and day
- Weather
- Pollution levels
- Age
- Skin colour
- Clothing
- Activity
- Amount of exposed skin
- Darker skin reduces vitamin D production from sunlight
- Sunscreen with a sun protection factor of 15 or more can completely inhibit vitamin D synthesis

Food

Few food types include vitamin D
Food provides a minimal contribution to overall vitamin D levels (176 IU–236 IU per day). Useful food types:

- Milk
- Margarine
- Fatty fish

Other issues

- Excessive amount of body fat. Obese individuals have less vitamin D bioavailability as vitamin D is stored in body fat
- Caffeine–4 cups of coffee a day is associated with hip fractures in men and women
- Alcohol–3 standard drinks per day consistently
- Sodium–higher sodium increases calcium excretion
- Smoking–any levels

surprisingly, smoking and excess alcohol intake are relatively weak risk factors, whereas a previous fracture or a family history of hip fracture are much stronger risk factors (University of Sheffield, 2018). As with other serious pathologies, careful history-taking is essential to identify all risk factors.

Osteoporosis can remain pain free for many years as the disease quietly progresses. There are often no symptoms relating to osteoporosis at all until bones actually fracture. Diagnosis of osteoporosis is often not made until a low-impact fracture has occurred. In fact, even when symptomatic, it is estimated that only one in three vertebral fractures come to clinical attention (International Osteoporosis Foundation, 2017). However, much can be done prophylactically to reduce the chances of osteoporosis developing in the first place; ideally osteoporosis risk should be identified prior to a fracture occurring. From a physiotherapy perspective, we have a huge role to play long before the disease becomes problematic. Physiotherapists should incorporate public health interventions such as Making Every Contact Count (MECC) (National Health Service (NHS) Public Health England, 2016) when working with younger patients and clients by including appropriate advice to those in their late teens to their mid-twenties when peak bone mass is achieved (see Chapter 4). Equally, in patients presenting with low trauma fracture, we have a duty of care to signpost to those experts who may optimise bone health. Initially, this is likely to be in the hands of the general practitioner, with more advanced cases needing the help of bone health experts including endocrinologists.

Why wait to help until years later when the Blue Light may need to be on?

Diagnosis of osteoporosis

Only once other forms of serious pathologies, such as myeloma, osteomalacia and hyperparathyroidism, have been excluded should osteoporosis be confirmed (Box 3.3).

The World Health Organization (WHO) defines osteoporosis based on BMD. A dual-energy x-ray absorptiometry (DEXA) scan is commonly used to diagnose osteoporosis before a fracture occurs and helps to estimate future risk of low trauma fracture. A DEXA scan is a short painless procedure with lower radiation levels than traditional x-ray (NHS Choices, 2016), estimated to be a radiation dose equal to just one day in the sun (Arthritis Research UK, 2018). A DEXA scan provides a number of results used to inform bone health and fracture risk (Osteopenia and Osteoporosis Treatments and Cures; National Osteoporosis Foundation, 2017):

- BMD
- T score: BMD compared to peak bone mass age of young healthy women (i.e. thirties)
- Z score: BMD compared with that of same age population

The WHO T-score >2.5 standard deviations (SDs) identified on a DEXA scan is a well-recognised threshold for the diagnosis of and intervention in osteoporosis (Table 3.1). However, the majority of osteoporotic fractures actually occur in an osteopenic range where the T-score is less than −1 SD and greater than −2.5 SD.

▌BOX 3.3 Signs and symptoms of myeloma, osteomalacia and hyperparathyroidism.

Myeloma

The most common signs and symptoms of multiple myeloma (The Health line.com, 2018) include:

- Fatigue
- Bone pain
- Kidney problems
- Low blood count
- Frequent infections

Other common signs and symptoms of multiple myeloma include:

- Nausea
- Weight loss
- Constipation
- Loss of appetite
- Weakness or loss of feeling in legs
- Swelling in legs
- Increased thirst
- Frequent urination
- Dizziness
- Confusion
- Pain, especially in back or abdomen

Osteomalacia

(Mayo Clinic, 2017)

Dull, aching bone pain

- Lower back
- Pelvis
- Hips
- Legs
- Ribs

The pain might be worse at night, or when there is pressure on the bones, rarely relieved completely by rest

▍ BOX 3.3 Signs and symptoms of myeloma, osteomalacia and hyperparathyroidism.—cont'd

Muscle weakness
- Decreased muscle tone can cause a waddling gait and make walking slower and more difficult

Hyperparathyroidism
(BMJ Best Practice, 2018)

Key diagnostic factors
- Family history of hyperparathyroidism or features suggestive of hyperkalaemia
- Nephrolithiasis (kidney stones)
- History of osteoporosis or osteopenia

Other diagnostic factors
- Bone pain
- Poor sleep
- Fatigue
- Anxiety

Risk factors
- History of head and neck irradiation
- Female sex
- Age 50 to 60 years
- Family history of primary hyperparathyroidism

Prompted by national or local protocols, or by identification of risk factors, investigations into bone health should take place to establish the diagnosis of osteoporosis based on quantitative assessment of BMD (National Osteoporosis Guideline Group (NOGG), 2014). It is important to note that intervention thresholds can differ from diagnostic thresholds for a variety of reasons

TABLE 3.1 WHO definitions of bone mineral density levels based on DEXA measurements of hip, spine and forearm. Criteria for white postmenopausal women only (4bonehealth, 2018).

Definition	Criteria
Normal	Within +1 or −1 SD
Osteopenia (low bone mass)	Between −1 and −2.5 SD below young adult mean
Osteoporosis	≥ −2.5 SD below young adult mean
Severe osteoporosis	≥ −2.5 SD plus history of one or more osteoporotic fractures

DEXA, Dual-energy x-ray absorptiometry; *SD*, standard deviation; *WHO*, World Health Organization.

(National Institute for Health and Care Excellence (NICE), 2012). For instance, fracture risk is influenced by age even if there is an identical T-score. The UK-based NOGG group provides a number of aims relating to detailed examination and investigations listed below. It also provides helpful recommendations relating to which investigations should be considered (NOGG, 2014) (Boxes 3.4 & 3.5).

Investigations into bone health commonly combine the use of tools such as the fracture risk assessment tool (FRAX) (University of Sheffield, 2018) and DEXA. The FRAX tool can be used to assess the need for a DEXA scan. Alternatively, the FRAX tool can use the DEXA femoral neck BMD T-score to calculate fracture risk (Table 3.2).

▌BOX 3.4 NOGG (2014) suggested routine investigations for diagnosing osteoporosis.

Subjective and objective examination
Full blood count, erythrocyte sedimentation rate or C-reactive protein, serum calcium, albumin, creatinine, phosphate, alkaline phosphate, liver transaminases
Thyroid function tests
DEXA

▌BOX 3.5 NOGG (2014) identification of other suggested investigations which may be indicated. These and further tests are often carried out by specialist departments.

Lateral x-ray of lumbar and thoracic spine
Protein immunoelectrophoresis and urine Bence-Jones protein
25 OHD (25-hydroxycholecalciferol, or 25-hydroxyvitamin D: a prehormone that is produced in the liver by hydroxylation of vitamin D3)
PTH (parathyroid hormone)
Serum testosterone
Serum prolactin
24-hour urine cortisol/dexamethasone suppression test
Endomysial and/or tissue transglutaminase antibodies (coeliac disease)
Isotope bone scan
Markers of bone turnover
Urinary calcium excretion

As with most health conditions, there are a number of red herrings and comorbidities associated with low BMD that can ultimately lead to osteoporosis and to which clinicians should remain vigilant (Box 3.6).

▌TABLE 3.2 Methods to calculate fracture risk.

FRAX (age range 40–90 years)	Estimates 10-year predicted absolute fracture risk. Interpret those over 80 years with caution as short-term risk may be underestimated
DEXA	If bone mineral density found within threshold of intervention

DEXA, Dual-energy x-ray absorptiometry; *FRAX*, fracture risk assessment tool.

Fracture risk

Risk of osteoporotic fracture should not be underestimated. For the year 2000, there were an estimated nine million new osteoporotic fractures (International Osteoporosis Foundation, 2017), with the most common osteoporotic fracture sites being:

- wrist (1.7 million)
- hip (1.6 million)
- vertebrae (1.4 million)

With life expectancy increasing, it is estimated that over the next few decades fracture rates will rise by two or three times (International Osteoporosis Foundation, 2017). Hip fractures in particular significantly affect mortality.

Kanis et al. (2012) report 10-fold differences between countries in the risk of hip fracture and in the 10-year fracture probability worldwide (Table 3.3).

It is interesting to question why fracture risk varies so much internationally. The reasons are not completely clear. The patterns suggest that environmental rather than genetic factors are important (Kanis et al., 2012). This is supported by changes observed in the

BOX 3.6 Red herrings and comorbidities associated with low BMD (Hagen, 2011).

Comorbidities associated with reduced BMD

- Rheumatoid arthritis, lupus, vasculitis
- Chronic malnutrition or malabsorption: coeliac disease
- Crohn's disease
- Asthma, chronic obstructive pulmonary disease
- Chronic liver disease
- Chronic kidney failure
- Endocrine disease especially Cushing's, primary hyperparathyroidism, hyperthyroidism, hypogonadism, diabetes mellitus type 1
- Organ transplantation
- Menopause before age 45 years
- Anorexia/amenorrhea
- Neurological degenerative disease: multiple sclerosis, Parkinson's
- Chronic inflammatory conditions (e.g. inflammatory bowel disease)

Drugs associated with reduced BMD

- Thyroid hormone
- Warfarin
- Heparin
- Glucocorticoid >3 months in prior year (Prednisolone equivalent dose >7.5 mg)
- Drugs that induce hypogonadal state (e.g. tamoxifen, aromatase inhibitors)
- Androgen deprivation therapy
- Cytotoxic drugs (e.g. methotrexate)
- Lithium
- Proton pump inhibitors
- Antiepileptics
- Medroxyprogesterone acetate
- Selective serotonin reuptake inhibitors
- Cancer chemotherapeutic drugs
- Thiazolidinediones

TABLE 3.3 Variations in international hip fracture risk (Kanis et al., 2012).

High-Risk Countries/Regions	
North Western Europe	**Central and Southern Europe**
Iceland	Belgium
Ireland	Germany
Finland	Austria
Denmark	Switzerland
Sweden	Greece
Norway	Hungary
Eastern Europe	Czech Republic
Russian Federation	Slovakia
	Iran
	Kuwait
	Oman

Moderate-Risk Countries/Regions
Oceania
China
India
Argentina
Countries of North America

Low-Risk Countries/Regions
Latin America with the exception of Argentina
Africa
Saudi Arabia
Iberian Peninsula
Indonesia
Thailand

levels of risk in immigrant populations. For example, African Americans in the USA have lower fracture probabilities than Caucasians, but the incidence of hip fracture in US Blacks is much higher than in African Blacks.

Similar patterns are present in the Japanese population of Hawaii and among the Chinese population living in Hong Kong and Singapore compared with mainland China. One of the important environmental factors appears to be calcium nutrition. Paradoxically, in countries with higher calcium intake, there is greater hip fracture risk (Kanis et al., 2012) (Table 3.3). The age- and sex-specific incidence of fracture is changing around the world. Studies in Western populations generally report increases in hip fracture incidence throughout the second half of the 20th century, but those rates stabilised, and even decreased in some centres at the start of the 21st century. In other countries (for example, Japan, China, Turkey and Mexico), age-adjusted hip fracture rates continue to rise (Kanis et al., 2012).

With respect to the spine, five clinical features have been found useful to raise or lower the probability of vertebral fracture (Henschke et al., 2008):

- age >50 years (likelihood ratio [LR] +=2.2, LR−=0.34)
- female (LR+=2.3, LR−=0.67)
- major trauma (LR+=12.8, LR−=0.37)
- pain and tenderness (LR+=6.7, LR−=0.44)
- a distracting painful injury (LR+=1.7, LR−=0.78)

The FRAX tool was a major development in 2008 and is now used worldwide. This tool was developed using international data collection involving more than one million patient years of follow-up. FRAX allows the identification in a primary care setting of those at risk of osteoporosis and it estimates the 10-year probability of fracture based on 11 risk factors plus BMD. Even in countries where appropriate imaging is unavailable it is widely applicable, available online and in many languages (University of Sheffield, 2018). However, the current version of FRAX does not include fall-related risk, which is a strong risk factor of fracture.

Canadian guidelines recommend that all individuals over 50 years of age be tested for fragility fracture risk (Whelan et al., 2011). However, in the UK, NICE (2012) has adopted a different approach. NICE suggest that it is not appropriate to risk assess individuals randomly for fracture risk (Box 3.7). Instead, a process of clinical and hypothetical deductive reasoning should guide the clinician towards onward assessment.

The variety of international osteoporosis management guidelines are in place to inform clinical practice bespoke to the local population being treated. Fig. 3.2 is an example of a risk assessment and treatment pathway in a town in the North West of England. Note how management begins with lifestyle advice when risks are low and no Blue Light is on.

Before moving onto the next chapter, in which management of osteoporosis is discussed, let us revisit Marjorie (the woman we introduced at the beginning of this chapter). You will remember that she did not recall having ever received any advice on bone health protection when she was younger. She is now facing an emergency Blue Light situation. Let's move back in time to 1962 when Marjorie was 20 years old. Marjorie was a bookish girl, a dedicated follower of fashion, who did not like exercise. In keeping with her peer group, Marjorie maintained a low body weight and cultivated a pale complexion by staying out of the sun. Socially, Marjorie enjoyed evenings out with her friends smoking and drinking in local pubs. Hearing this history today should raise your

> **BOX 3.7** Osteoporosis: fragility fracture risk (NICE, 2012).
>
> 1. Consider assessment of fracture risk:
>   - in all women aged 65 years and over and all men aged 75 years and over
>   - in women aged under 65 years and men aged under 75 years in the presence of specific risk factors, e.g.:
>   - previous fragility fracture
>   - current use or frequent recent use of oral or systemic glucocorticoids
>   - history of falls
>   - family history of hip fracture
>   - other causes of secondary osteoporosis
>   - low body mass index (BMI) (less than 18.5 kg/m^2)
>   - smoking
>   - alcohol intake of more than 14 units per week for women and more than 21 units per week for men.
> 2. Do not routinely assess fracture risk in people aged under 50 years unless they have major risk factors, e.g.:
>   - current or frequent recent use of oral or systemic glucocorticoids
>   - untreated premature menopause
>   - previous fragility fracture.

index of suspicion that Marjorie is at high risk of developing osteoporosis later in life. The next chapter will provide you with advice and strategies that may be relevant to help you to help the next 'young Marjorie' who walks into your clinic.

Osteoporosis/fracture risk assessment & treatment pathway

Any patient that presents with a fragility fracture should be classed as high risk

If risks concern you, assess a patients FRAX score via
https://www.sheffield.ac.uk/FRAX/tool.jsp

Increased risk of osteoporosis occurs
in patients with the following:
- women 65 years and older
- men 75 years and older
- BMI less than 18.5 kg/m2
- 3 months or more steroid use

Over 50s with

- oral steroids
- parent history of hip fracture
- smoker or high alcohol intake

Under 50s with

- untreated menopause

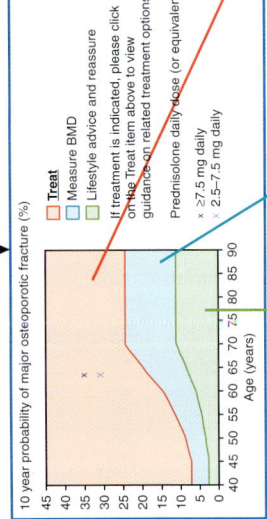

10 year probability of major osteoporotic fracture (%)

Treat

Measure BMD

Lifestyle advice and reassure

If treatment is indicated, please click
on the Treat item above to view
guidance on related treatment options.

Prednisolone daily dose (or equivalent)

× ≥7.5 mg daily
× 2.5–7.5 mg daily

Age (years)

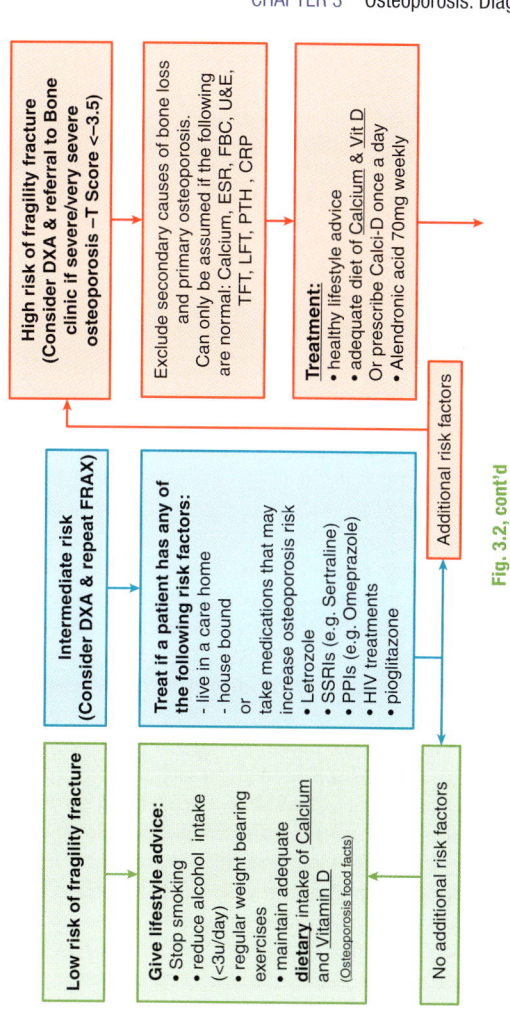

High risk of fragility fracture
(Consider DXA & referral to Bone clinic if severe/very severe osteoporosis −T Score <−3.5)

Exclude secondary causes of bone loss and primary osteoporosis.
Can only be assumed if the following are normal: Calcium, ESR, FBC, U&E, TFT, LFT, PTH , CRP

Treatment:
• healthy lifestyle advice
• adequate diet of Calcium & Vit D
Or prescribe Calci-D once a day
• Alendronic acid 70mg weekly

Intermediate risk
(Consider DXA & repeat FRAX)

Treat if a patient has any of the following risk factors:
- live in a care home
- house bound
or
take medications that may increase osteoporosis risk
• Letrozole
• SSRIs (e.g. Sertraline)
• PPIs (e.g. Omeprazole)
• HIV treatments
• pioglitazone

Additional risk factors

Low risk of fragility fracture

Give lifestyle advice:
• Stop smoking
• reduce alcohol intake (<3u/day)
• regular weight bearing exercises
• maintain adequate **dietary** intake of <u>Calcium</u> and <u>Vitamin D</u>
(Osteoporosis food facts)

No additional risk factors

Fig. 3.2, cont'd

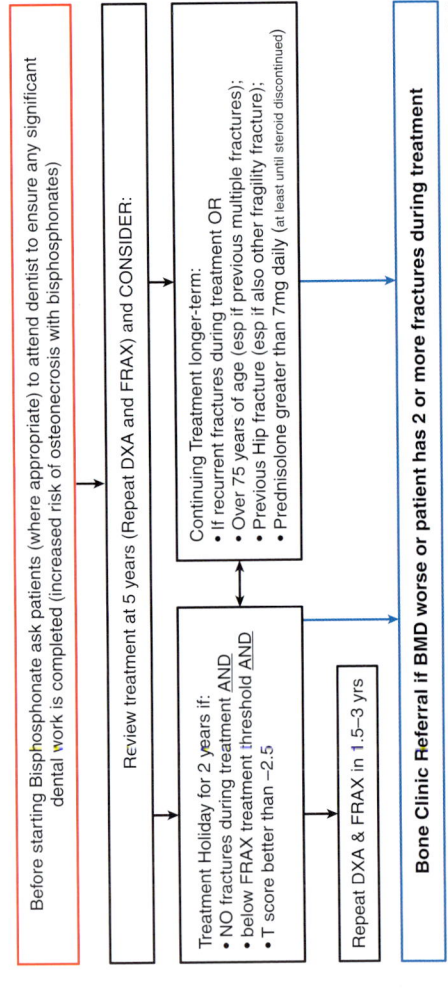

Before starting Bisphosphonate ask patients (where appropriate) to attend dentist to ensure any significant dental work is completed (increased risk of osteonecrosis with bisphosphonates)

Review treatment at 5 years (Repeat DXA and FRAX) and CONSIDER:

Continuing Treatment longer-term:
• If recurrent fractures during treatment OR
• Over 75 years of age (esp if previous multiple fractures);
• Previous Hip fracture (esp if also other fragility fracture);
• Prednisolone greater than 7mg daily (at least until steroid discontinued)

Treatment Holiday for 2 years if:
• NO fractures during treatment AND
• below FRAX treatment threshold AND
• T score better than −2.5

Repeat DXA & FRAX in 1.5–3 yrs

Bone Clinic Referral if BMD worse or patient has 2 or more fractures during treatment

Fig. 3.2 Example of a local osteoporosis/fracture risk assessment & treatment pathway. *BMD,* Bone mineral density; *BMI,* body mass index; *CRP,* C-reactive protein; *DXA,* dual-energy x-ray absorptiometry; *ESR,* erythrocyte sedimentation rate; *FBC,* full blood count; *FRAX* fracture risk assessment tool; *LFT,* liver function test; *PPI,* proton-pump inhibitor; *PTH,* parathyroid hormone; *SSRI,* selective serotonin reuptake inhibitor; *TFT,* thyroid function test; *U&E,* urea and electrolytes.

References

4bone health. Criteria for diagnosing osteoporosis. 2018. http://www.4bonehealth.org/education/world-health-organization-criteria-diagnosis-osteoporosis/.

Arthritis Research UK. 2018. https://www.arthritisresearchuk.org/arthritis-information/conditions/osteoporosis/diagnosis.aspx.

BMJ Best Practice. Primary hyperparathyroidism. 2018. http://bestpractice.bmj.com/topics/en-gb/133.

Bolton CCG. (2018) Osteoporosis Pathway 2018. Authors: Medicines Optimisation & Dept of Rheumatology Review date: February 2021.

Bombak A, Hanson H. Qualitative insights from the osteoporosis research: a narrative review of the literature. *J Osteoporos*. 2016. www.ncbi.nlm.nih.gov.

Cooper C, Harvey N. (2012). BMJ 2012;344:e4191.

Gosch M, Kammerlander C, Nicholas J. Treatment of osteoporosis in older adults. *Panminerva Med*. 2014;56(2):133–143. E pub.

Greenhalgh S, Selfe J. Screen for red flags first: don't take the bio out of biopsychosocial. In: Porter S, ed. *Psychologically Informed Physiotherapy*. Elsevier; 2017.

Hagen S. Osteoporosis: Nutrition and lifestyle. *Canadian Pharmacist Journal*. 2011. Available on: http://journals.sagepub.com/doi/abs/10.3821/1913-701X-144.SUPPL1.S14.

Harding M. Osteoporosis. 2017. https://patient.info/health/osteoporosis-leaflet.

Hartvigsen J, Hancock M, Kongsted A, et al. Low back pain 1: what low back pain is and why we need to pay attention. Lancet Low Back Pain Series Working Group. *Lancet*. 2018. https://doi.org/10.1016/s0140-6736(18)30480-X.

Henschke N, Maher CG, Refshauge KM. A systematic review identifies five "red flags" to screen for vertebral fracture in patients with low back pain. *J Clin Epidemiol*. 2008;61(2):110–118.

International Osteoporosis Foundation. Facts and Statistics; 2017. https://www.iofbonehealth.org/facts-statistics.

Ito M, Yamad M, Hayashi K, et al. Relation of early menarche to high bone mineral density. *Calcif Tissue Int*. 1995;57(1):11–14.

Kanis JA, Odén A, McCloskey EV, et al. A systematic review of hip fracture incidence and probability of fracture worldwide. *Osteoporos Int*. 2012;23(9):2239–2256.

Mayo Clinic. Osteomalacia. Symptoms and Causes. 2017. https://www. mayoclinic.org/diseases-conditions/osteomalacia/symptoms-causes/ syc-20355514.

National Institute of Arthritis and Musculoskeletal and Skin Diseases. Osteoporosis. 2016. https://www.niams.nih.gov/health-topics/osteoporosis#tab-causes.

National Osteoporosis Foundation. Bone Density Exam/testing; 2017. https://www.nof.org/patients/diagnosis-information/bone-density-examtesting/.

National Osteoporosis Guideline Group (NOGG). Guideline for the diagnosis and management of osteoporosis in postmenopausal women and men from the age of 50 years in the UK. 2014. https://www.sheffield. ac.uk/NOGG/NOGG%20Guideline%202017.pdf.

National Osteoporosis Society. The Osteoporosis Agenda England. 2015. Available at: https://theros.org.uk/media/1959/agenda-for-osteoporosis-england-final.pdf.

National Osteoporosis Society. Are you at risk? 2018. Available on: https://www.nof.org/preventing-fractures/general-facts/bone-basics/are-you-at-risk/.

NHS Choices. DEXA (DXA) scan. 2016. https://www.nhs.uk/conditions/ DEXA-scan/.

NHS Public Health England. Making Every Contact Count (MECC): Consensus statement Produced by Public Health England. NHS England and Health Education England, April 2016; 2016.

NICE. Osteoporosis: assessing the risk of fragility fracture (CG146). 2012. https://www.nice.org.uk/guidance/cg146/chapter/1-Guidance.

Osteopenia and Osteopxorosis Treatments and Cures. Understanding your DEXA scan results. http://www.osteopenia3.com/dexascan. html.

Premkumar A, Godfrey W, Gottschalk M, Boden S. Red flags for low back pain are not always really red. *J Bone Joint Surg Am*. 2018;100:368–374.

Ross AC, Taylor CL, Yaktine AL, et al. Institute of Medicine (US) Committee to Review Dietary Reference Intakes for Vitamin D and Calcium. Washington (DC): National Academies Press (US); 2011.

The Health line.com. Signs and Symptoms of Multiple Myeloma. 2018. https://www.healthline.com/health/cancer/multiple-myeloma-signs-symptoms#symptoms.

University of Sheffield. FRAX® Fracture Risk Assessment Tool. 2018. http://www.shef.ac.uk/FRAX/.

Weaver C, Gordon C, Janz K, et al. The National Osteoporosis Foundation's position statement on peak bone mass development and lifestyle factors: a systematic review and implementation recommendations. *Osteopros Int.* 2016;144:S4–S4. Available at: https://www.ncbi.nlm.nih.gov/pmc/articles/PMC4791473/.

Whelan A. Osteoporosis care gap: an opportunity for primary health care practitioners. *Osteoporosis In Primary Care. Canadian Pharmacist Journal*; 2011.

CHAPTER 4

Osteoporosis: Consequences and Care

This chapter concentrates on the use of prophylaxis to help patients such as the young Marjorie (see Chapter 3) rather than the complex care of advanced osteoporosis needed in the case of older Marjorie, which we will leave to the specialist care of bone health experts. Physiotherapists have a crucial role to play from many perspectives in osteoporosis prophylaxis to prevent the Blue Light condition from developing in later years.

To reduce the impact of osteoporosis, the National Osteoporosis Foundation (2014) has listed universal recommendations to guide healthcare consultations. Some of these are:

- advice on the risk of osteoporosis and related fractures
- advice on a diet that includes adequate amounts of total calcium and vitamin D intake and incorporation of dietary supplements if diet is insufficient
- recommendations on regular weight-bearing and muscle-strengthening exercises to improve muscle strength, posture and balance; reduce the risk of falls and fractures; and maintain or improve bone strength
- assessment of risk factors for falls and offering appropriate modifications (e.g. home safety assessment, balance-training exercises)
- advice on cessation of tobacco smoking and avoidance of excessive alcohol intake

These universal recommendations fit well with the concept of 'Making Every Contact Count' (MECC), which is a public health approach being promoted in the UK (National Health Service (NHS), 2016). Launched in 2016, MECC is an approach to behaviour change that uses the millions of day-to-day interactions that organisations and people have with other people to support them in making positive changes to their physical and mental health and wellbeing. MECC encourages opportunistic delivery of concise healthy lifestyle information and enables individuals to engage in conversations about their health. In particular, MECC maximises the opportunity within routine health and care interactions for a brief or very brief discussion on health or wellbeing factors to take place. MECC interactions take just a few minutes and are not intended to add to the existing workloads of healthcare staff; they aim to fit into and complement existing clinical approaches. In the UK, physiotherapists are being encouraged to adopt MECC to help people make healthier choices to achieve positive long-term change in behaviour, in addition to focusing solely on the presenting health problem. If a physiotherapist chooses to take on this wider public health role as advocated by the MECC approach, and is asking a patient to change their behaviour, Michie et al. (2011) suggest that patients must have the:

- capability—both physically and psychologically
- opportunity—both physical opportunity (space, equipment, time, etc.), and social opportunity (within family, social environment)
- motivation—self-efficacy, perception of positive benefits, desire to overcome inhibitive habits (Fig. 4.1)

As this is a relatively new approach in physiotherapy practice, these three domains of capability, opportunity

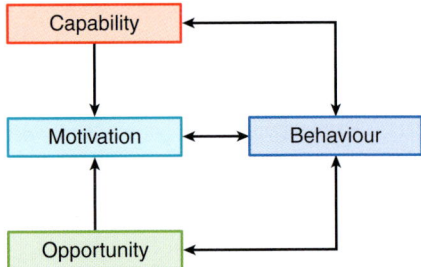

Fig. 4.1 COM-B model adapted from Michie et al. (2011).

and motivation are not always systematically addressed during consultations. It is therefore possible that physiotherapists, who are potentially key professionals in delivering wider public health and lifestyle messages, are not currently maximising the potential benefits of MECC (Michie et al., 2011).

Osteoporotic fractures

Risk factors of falls (Hagan, 2011):
- biological—poor balance affecting gait, visual, hearing impaired, medical condition
- medication—four or more (polypharmacy), side effects
- environmental—hazards
- socioeconomical—living alone, isolation, weak family support
- behavioural—fear avoidant, excess alcohol, clothing, walking aid

Fractures and their complications are common clinical consequences of osteoporosis. In the USA, two million fractures are attributed annually to osteoporosis, causing more than 432,000 hospital admissions, almost 2.5 million doctor consultations and approximately 180,000 nursing home admissions (Office of the Surgeon General, 2004). Due in part to an ageing population, the cost of care for osteoporosis is expected to rise to $25.3 billion by 2025 (Burge et al., 2007). A low-energy fracture is usually defined as a fracture resulting from minimal trauma incurred due to falling from standing height or less (Cooper & Melton, 1996). It is unlikely a healthy individual would sustain a fracture as a consequence of such a fall. There is always a need to discriminate between an osteoporotic fragility fracture and a fracture caused by malignancy such as myeloma or spinal metastases. A recent fracture at any major skeletal site in an adult older than 50 years of age should be considered a significant event for the diagnosis of osteoporosis. Apart from pain and dysfunction, fractures can also cause psychosocial symptoms, most notably depression and loss of self-esteem which often occur due to loss of independence (National Osteoporosis Foundation, 2014).

Older adults with learning difficulties make up a distinct population group who suffer disproportionately high rates of osteoporotic fractures, as the number of individuals with complex learning and physical difficulties surviving to older age is increasing. Morbidity after fracture is also likely to be more serious in this population. This is a relatively new phenomenon as adults with complex health needs and learning disabilities have not historically lived to older ages (Hubert & Hollins, 2000). (Tannenbaum et al., 1989) report that fractures occur 1.7–3.5 times more frequently in people with intellectual disabilities than in the general population. Health problems such as epilepsy and anticonvulsant medications are associated with the development of osteoporosis (Srikanth et al., 2011), poor diet, reduced mobility and weight bearing; these factors also predispose adults with learning disabilities to low bone density and falls. One of the things we have emphasised throughout this book is that the subjective examination is vitally important in establishing whether a patient may have a serious pathology. However, there are often significant challenges in communicating with adults with learning disabilities which may prevent the physiotherapist from gaining a clear history of the mechanism of injury or even establishing the exact site of pain.

For the year 2000, there were an estimated 9 million new osteoporotic fractures (International Osteoporosis Foundation, 2017) with the most common osteoporotic fracture sites being:

- wrist (1.7 million)
- hip (1.6 million)
- vertebrae (1.4 million)

Wrist fractures

Overall, although the most common, wrist fractures are probably the least disabling. However, they can interfere with activities of daily living such as dressing, washing and the preparation and eating of food. In the UK, there is often a peak in elderly patients being referred for physiotherapy around the month of March as this is typically when people who have slipped on ice in January have their plaster casts or splints removed.

Hip fractures

Hip fractures are associated with an 8.4% to 36% excess mortality within 1 year, with a higher mortality rate in men than in women (Office of the Surgeon General, 2004). Hip fractures are associated with a 2.5 times increased risk of future fractures (Colón-Emeric et al., 2003). Approximately

20% of hip fracture patients require long-term nursing home care, and only 40% fully regain their pre-fracture level of independence (Lewiecki & Laster, 2006).

Vertebral fractures

Although the majority of vertebral fractures are initially clinically silent, these fractures are often later associated with symptoms of pain, disability, deformity and mortality (Abrahamsen et al., 2009). Underdiagnosis of vertebral fracture is a worldwide problem. The proportion of vertebral fractures that go unrecognised during the local assessment of a thoracolumbar lateral radiograph is as high as 46% in Latin America, 45% in North America and 29% in Europe/South Africa/Australia (International Osteoporosis Foundation, 2017). Postural changes associated with kyphosis may limit activity, including bending and reaching. Multiple thoracic fractures may result in restrictive lung disease and lumbar fractures, which may alter abdominal anatomy, leading to constipation, abdominal pain, distention, reduced appetite and premature satiety. Vertebral fractures, whether clinically apparent or silent, are major predictors of future fracture risk, and result in up to 5 times greater risk for subsequent vertebral fracture and 2 to 3 times greater risk for fractures at other sites (National Osteoporosis Foundation, 2014). Roman et al. (2010) retrospectively analysed 1448 patients who attended a tertiary care spinal surgery centre between 2005 and 2009. Thirty-eight patients (2.6%) with a spinal osteoporotic fracture were identified. The authors combined 56 clinical Red Flags to form a 5-item diagnostic decision model:

- age <22 or >52 years
- low body mass index (BMI)

- female gender
- no presence of leg pain
- does not exercise regularly

Having only 2 out of 5 features yielded a negative likelihood ratio of 0.16 (95% CI = 0.04–0.51) and it therefore seemed informative to rule out the presence of a spinal fracture. On the other hand, having 4 out of 5 items resulted in a positive likelihood ratio of 9.6 (95% CI = 3.7–14.9) which increased the post-test probability up to 20% of suffering from an osteoporotic vertebral fracture (based on a pre-test probability of 2.6% within the study cohort). The post-fracture osteoporosis care gap is currently often a missed opportunity in primary care. A Canadian study identified that only 1 out of 5 women with osteoporotic-related fractures were investigated and/or offered treatment for osteoporosis, leaving them at 4 to 5 times higher risk of future fragility fractures (Whelan, 2011). Post-fracture nutrition is important for at least 6 out of 12 patients after fracture (Hagan, 2011). Specific nutrients that need to be considered are:

- calcium
- vitamin D
- protein
- calories
- vitamin B12
- folate

Vitamin D

Vitamin D is very important as it plays a major role in calcium absorption, bone health, muscle performance, balance and risk of falling (National Osteoporosis Foundation, 2014).

Many older patients are at high risk for vitamin D deficiency, including:

- patients with malabsorption or other intestinal diseases
- chronic renal insufficiency
- patients on medications that increase the breakdown of vitamin D (e.g. some anti-seizure drugs)
- housebound patients
- chronically ill patients
- those with limited sun exposure
- individuals with very dark skin
- obese individuals

Physiotherapy

In the UK, an increasing number of physiotherapists are becoming independent prescribers. Issues relating to polypharmacy are important in fall prevention. Reducing or eliminating unnecessary medication from an individual's medication regime is as important as prescribing the correct medication for a specific set of symptoms. Drug regimens are only briefly mentioned, and an exhaustive discussion of these will not be presented. Physiotherapists working in specialist roles in relation to osteoporosis should find other sources of detailed information relating to current pharmaceutical approaches to the management of osteoporosis. Basic pharmacological treatment of osteoporosis usually requires supplementation of calcium and vitamin D each day (Gosch et al., 2014).

Gosch et al. (2014) list the following as important pharmaceutical agents to be considered in the treatment of osteoporosis:

- hormone therapy in postmenopausal women
- bisphosphonates
- denosumab

- strontium ranelate
- parathyroid hormone (PTH) and teriparatide

Following the MECC approach, physiotherapists should be recommending regular weight-bearing and muscle-strengthening exercises to help reduce the risk of falls and fractures (Sherrington et al., 2008; Choi & Hector, 2012; Gillespie et al., 2012; Granacher et al., 2013). Among the wider health benefits, weight-bearing and muscle-strengthening exercises can also improve agility, strength, posture and balance, which may reduce the risk of falls. In addition, exercise may modestly increase bone density. Physical activity should be encouraged in all age groups, both for osteoporosis prevention and overall health, as the benefits of exercise are lost when people stop exercising. NHS Choices in the UK also recommends regular exercise. Current guidance suggests adults aged 19 to 64 should do at least 150 minutes (2 hours and 30 minutes) of moderate-intensity aerobic activity, such as cycling or fast walking, every week. Weight-bearing exercise and resistance exercise are particularly important for improving bone density and helping to prevent osteoporosis. In addition to aerobic exercise, adults aged 19 to 64 should also do muscle-strengthening activities on two or more days a week by working all the major muscle groups, including the legs, hips, back, abdomen, chest, shoulders and arms. Physiotherapists should complement any exercise programmes with additional advice regarding measures which patients can take to reduce the risk of falls. For example, checking their homes for trip hazards, such as trailing wires, making sure rugs and carpets are secure and keeping rubber mats by the sink and in the bath to prevent slipping.

The CSP (2017; Box 4.1) and the National Osteoporosis Foundation (2003) provides a comprehensive list of activities that physiotherapists could address during consultations:

- Avoid long-term immobilisation and recommend partial bed rest (with periodic sitting and ambulating) only when required and for the shortest periods possible
- Proper exercise may improve physical performance/ function, bone mass, muscle strength and balance, and reduce the risk of falling
- Walking and daily activities, such as housework and gardening, are practical ways to contribute to maintenance of fitness and bone mass
- Improve posture and balance; advise patients to avoid forward bending and exercising with the trunk in flexion during balance training, especially in combination with twisting
- Strengthen quadriceps through progressive resistance training to allow a person to rise unassisted from a chair
- Stretch tight soft tissues and joints
- If appropriate, promote use of assistive devices to help with ambulation, balance, lifting and reaching
- Assess home environment for risk factors for falls and intervene as appropriate
- In patients with acute vertebral fractures or chronic pain due to multiple vertebral fractures, the use of trunk orthoses (e.g. back brace, corset and posture-training support devices) may provide pain relief by reducing the loads on the fracture sites and aligning the vertebrae. However, long-term bracing may lead to muscle weakness and further deconditioning

The National Osteoporosis Society (2014) also provides a useful framework for exercise prescription in osteoporosis, where they categorise people into exercise groups for low risk of fracture, high risk of fracture and stability and balance (fall prevention).

Suggested exercises for people with low risk of fracture

- Jumping/bouncing on the spot

  Start with just three to five small, low jumps for the first few sessions. Build up gradually by adding five jumps at a time. Progress until the person can do 50 in total. Make sure participants take a brief rest between each set of 10 repetitions and pause briefly between each jump. Build up to 50 jumps a day that lift feet 7–8 cm (approximately 3 inches) off the floor.

- Skipping for a few minutes daily is also a good impact exercise that will benefit bone health
- Intermittent jogging is a good exercise for people who find continuous jogging too strenuous, and involves alternate jogging and walking every 20 metres or so
- A combination of stair-climbing and intermittent jogging is good for improving bone density in the spine and hip in older women
- Dancing

Suggested exercises for people with high risk of fracture

Avoid

High-impact, fast-moving exercises such as jumping, running, jogging or skipping. Avoid jerky, rapid movements in general. Exercises in which participants are required to bend forwards and twist their waist, such as touching toes or doing sit-ups, should also be avoided. Other activities that require bending or twisting forcefully at the waist are golf, tennis, bowling and some yoga poses. If your patients enjoy this type of activity, they may need to adapt their technique to avoid forward flexion rather than giving it up entirely.

Choose

Low-impact exercises with controlled movements such as side-stepping, knee-lifting and so on. Examples include walking, dancing, low-impact aerobics, elliptical (cross) training machines and stair climbing.

Stability and balance (fall prevention) exercises

Exercises that improve the strength of the quadriceps can also help to reduce the risk of falling. Simply performing sit-to-stand and stand-to-sit exercises from a chair can help to strengthen the thigh muscles if done regularly. There is also evidence that taking part in regular sessions of Tai Chi can help to reduce the risk of falls.

Tandem stand
- Stand sideways next to a wall and place one hand on it for support, if needed
- Place one foot directly in front of the other so that the heel of one foot is just touching the toes of the other foot, try to stay as still as possible for 10 seconds. Rest. Repeat five times

Tandem walk
- Use a wall for support if needed
- Place one foot in front of the other so that the heel of the forward foot touches the toes of the rear foot
- Move forwards as if on a tightrope with the heel of one foot touching the toes of the other for approximately 10 feet, repeat five times

▌ **BOX 4.1** Chartered Society of Physiotherapy top tips for osteoporosis (CSP, 2017).

- Weight-bearing exercise, such as walking, can help to strengthen bones
- Exercises to improve balance and strength will help to prevent falls
- Follow a healthy diet that includes enough calcium and vitamin D
- Use this handy calculator to make sure you are getting enough calcium http://www.rheum.med.ed.ac.uk/calcium-calculator.php
- Wear sensible, well-fitting shoes to avoid falls
- Avoid rugs and sloppy slippers—both can cause trips
- Have good lighting on your stairs
- Get your eyesight checked regularly (free for people over 60 in the UK)
- Try to avoid heavy lifting—consider home delivery grocery shopping

The National Osteoporosis Society (2014) presented the fracture liaison service (FLS) as a proven model and the best approach to prevent future fractures in 2015. These services target patients aged over 50 who present to a healthcare setting with a fracture. They claim that the connection between over 50s presenting with a fracture and osteoporosis is frequently missed. It is estimated that the FLS approach to early diagnosis could prevent approximately 20,000 hip fractures in the UK annually. Unfortunately, despite this proven approach, uptake in healthcare organisations is limited.

Returning to Marjorie, in light of Roman et al.'s (2010) diagnostic decision model:

- age <22 or >52 years
- low BMI
- female gender

- no presence of leg pain
- does not exercise regularly

At presentation, Marjorie had all five Red Flags (she was 75 years old, had a BMI of 19, was a female, had no leg pain and had never participated in any exercise), so what advice should we have given to Marjorie in 1962? Marjorie and her friends needed to become trendsetters, taking up dancing and exercise instead of continuing with their more sedentary hobbies. A healthier diet was essential, along with sensible exposure to sunlight. Admittedly, public health knowledge was less extensive and less readily available in 1962 compared with the wealth of information which is available now at the touch of a button. However, knowledge of the side effects of smoking and alcohol on bone health may have helped. Importantly, in 1962, we should have helped Marjorie by suggesting a lifestyle change which would impact on her bone health throughout the rest of her life. If we had, Marjorie may not have needed the Blue Light approach to her condition in 2018.

References

Abrahamsen B, van Staa T, Ariely R, Olson M, Cooper C. Excess mortality following hip fracture: a systematic epidemiological review. *Osteoporos Int.* 2009;20(10):1633–1650.

Burge R, Dawson-Hughes B, Solomon DH, Wong JB, King AB, Tosteson A. Incidence and economic burden of osteoporosis-related fractures in the United States, 2005-2025. *J Bone Min Res.* 2007;22(3):465–475.

Chartered Society of Physiotherapy (CSP). Osteoporosis Fact Sheet; 2017. http://www.csp.org.uk/your-health/conditions/osteoporosis#top-tips-osteoporosis.

Choi M, Hector M. Effectiveness of intervention programs in preventing falls: a systematic review of recent 10 years and meta-analysis. *J Am Med Dir Assoc.* 2012;13(2):188.e13–e21.

Colón-Emeric C, Kuchibhatla M, Pieper C, et al. The contribution of hip fracture to risk of subsequent fractures: data from two longitudinal studies. *Osteoporos Int.* 2003;11:879–883.

Cooper C, Melton LJ. *Magnitude and Impact of Osteoporosis and Fractures.* San Diego: Academic Press; 1996.

Gillespie LD, Robertson MC, Gillespie WJ, Sherrington C, Gates S, Clemson LM, Lamb SE. Interventions for preventing falls in older people living in the community. *Cochrane Database Syst Rev.* 2012;12(9):CD007146.

Gosch M, Kammerlander C, Nicholas J. Treatment of osteoporosis in older adults. *Panminerva Med.* 2014;56(2):133–143.

Granacher U, Gollhofer A, Hortobágyi T, Kressig RW, Muehlbauer T. The importance of trunk muscle strength for balance, functional performance and fall prevention in seniors: a systematic review. *Sports Med.* 2013;43(7):627–641.

Hagan S. Osteoporosis: nutrition and lifestyle. *Can Pharm J.* 2011;114(suppl 1):S14.

Hubert M, Hollins S. Working with elderly carers of people with learning difficulties and lanning for the future. *Adv Psychiatr Treat.* 2000;6:41–48.

International Osteoporosis Foundation. Facts and statistics. 2017. https://www.iofbonehealth.org/facts-statistics.

Lewiecki EM, Laster AJ. Clinical review: clinical applications of vertebral fracture assessment by dual-energy x-ray absorptiometry. *J Clin Endo Metab.* 2006;91(11):4215–4222.

Michie S, van Stralen M, West R. The behaviour change wheel: a new method for characterising and designing behaviour change interventions. *Implement Sci.* 2011;6(1):42.

National Osteoporosis Foundation. *Health Professional's Guide to Rehabilitation of the Patient with Osteoporosis.* Washington, DC: National Osteoporosis Foundation; 2003.

National Osteoporosis Foundation. *Clinician's Guide to Prevention and Treatment of Osteoporosis.* Washington, DC: National Osteoporosis Foundation; 2014.

National Osteoporosis Society. *Exercise and Osteoporosis.* Camerton: Bath BA2 0PJ; 2014.

NHS Public Health England. *Making Every Contact Count (MECC): Consensus Statement Produced by Public Health England.* NHS England and Health Education England, April 2016.

Office of the Surgeon General (US). *Bone Health and Osteoporosis: A Report of the Surgeon General.* Rockville (MD): Office of the Surgeon General (US); 2004. Available from: http://www.ncbi.nlm.nih.gov/books/NBK45513/.

Roman M, Brown C, Richardson W, et al. The development of a clinical decision-making algorithm for detection of osteoporotic compression fractures or wedge deformity. *J Man Manip Ther.* 2010;18(1):44–49.

Sherrington C, Whitney JC, Lord SR, Herbert RD, Cumming RG, Close JC. Effective exercise for the prevention of falls: a systematic review and meta-analysis. *J Am Geriatr Soc.* 2008;56(12):2234–2243.

Srikanth R, Cassidy G, Joiner C, Teeluckdharry S. Osteoporosis in people with intellectual disabilities: a review and a brief study of risk factors for osteoporosis in a community sample of people with intellectual disabilities. *J Intellect Disabil Res.* 2011;55(1):53–62.

Tannenbaum T, Lipworth L, Baker S. Risk of fractures in an intermediate care facility for persons with mental retardation. *Am J Ment Retard.* 1989;93:444–451.

Whelan A. Osteoporosis care gap: an opportunity for primary healthcare practitioners. *Can Pharm J.* 2011;114(suppl 1):S4.

CHAPTER 5

Cauda Equina Syndrome: Diagnosis

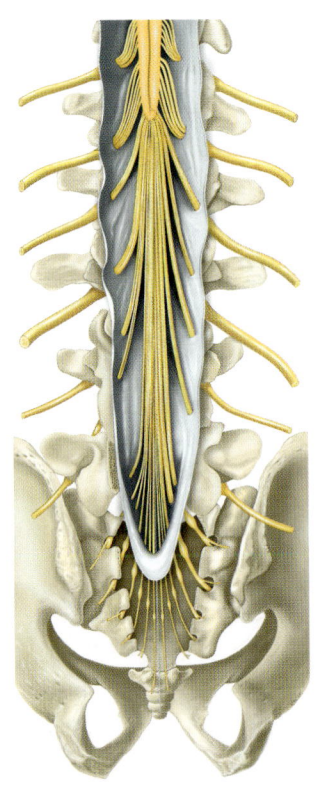

Introduction

At a time when the understanding of the link between lumbar disc herniation and cauda equina syndrome (CES) was in its infancy, Mennell (1952) discusses in some detail the importance of dysfunction of the genitourinary system as a potential cause of back pain and describes cases of the following:

- ischiorectal abscess (leading to death)
- carcinoma of the prostate
- kidney complaints (acute nephritis, renal calculus, moveable kidney)
- infection of the genitourinary system (bladder, cervix, gonorrhoea)
- uterine problems (fibroids, impacted pregnant uterus, prolapse or retroversion)
- haemorrhoids

Interestingly, however, Mennell does not mention intervertebral discs as a likely cause of CES. However, he does describe a case of a patient with Parkinson's disease who had long-standing back pain which was usually relieved by manipulation of the sacro-iliac junction. In this case, the previously successful treatment did not provide any relief and:

> Within two weeks sensory changes and loss of anal reflex set in. The patient had a minute tumour of the cauda equina… (p. 45)

By the time Cyriax was writing nearly a decade later in 1960, the disc as a cause of CES was well understood:

> Increased awareness of this syndrome among doctors should lead to a wider realization that there does exist a

dangerous form of lumbago, rare though its incidence is.
In these cases, we urge the patient to agree to laminectomy
before the development of the fourth sacral palsy.

What is particularly interesting from this extract is the call for a prophylactic laminectomy before it is too late! This is very much in tune with current guidelines.

Maitland (1977), Grieve (1979) and McKenzie (1981) all recognise the importance of CES and link it to herniated or protruding intervertebral discs. Grieve (1979) gives the most comprehensive guide to the identification of CES by suggesting that the following questions should be mandatory during the history-taking of a patient with pain in the lumbar region:

Any perineal or 'saddle area' anaesthesia or paraesthesia?

Any change in micturition habits associated with the back trouble, or sphincter disturbance? (p. 2)

A recent search on Google scholar revealed that there were 41,500 papers published with CES in the title. The number of papers published per decade throughout the 20th century increased slowly until the latter part of the century, with a massive rise in the number of papers being published in the first decade of the 21st century (Fig. 5.1).

The pattern of increased numbers of publications on CES is related to a number of factors associated with the digital information revolution that took place during the 1980s. This led to increasing opportunities for clinicians and academics to publish papers. It also meant it became much easier for patients to access information that would have previously only been available to medical

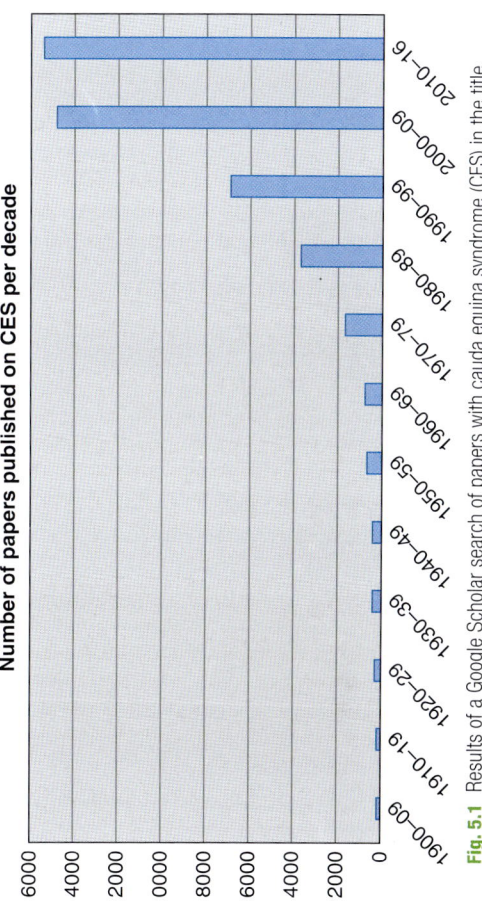

Fig. 5.1 Results of a Google Scholar search of papers with cauda equina syndrome (CES) in the title.

professionals. This potentially created an environment where an increasingly litigious culture became a further strong driver for clinicians and academics to publish in an attempt to safeguard themselves, thus contributing to the publishing boom. Price (2010) adds that, in the UK, this coincided with political changes from the 1980s to the end of the 20th century where the government initiated the gradual introduction of privatisation into the National Health Service (NHS), at a time when there was an increase in patients' expectations. Ethical issues, human rights, patients' rights and consumer expectations all converged during this time to exacerbate an increased use of litigation in cases of alleged medical negligence.

It is interesting to reflect that against this backdrop of increased numbers of publications and cases of litigation for CES, the number of actual CES cases has probably remained relatively static. CES is considered a rare condition occurring in less than 2% of all herniated discs, which, in view of the total number of episodes of low back pain (LBP) there are per year, remains a very small number. Gardner et al. (2011) estimated that in the UK there are just 30–40 cases of CES per year and Todd (2011) found that CES is more common in men. Todd (2011) highlights that the problems surrounding the identification and subsequent management of CES are probably not due to a lack of knowledge about CES, but probably more to do with a failure to apply a well-established knowledge base.

Three factors determine outcome in CES patients (Todd & Dickson, 2016):
- the degree of neurological deficit
- the duration of compression
- the speed of onset of the lesion

The worse the deficit, the longer the compression and the more rapid the onset of deficit, the worse the outcome (Fig. 5.2).

Anatomy of the cauda equina

The cauda equina was named after its resemblance to a horse's tail by the French anatomist André du Laurens in his book *Historia Anatomica Humani Corporis,* which was first published in Paris in 1600, (Du Laurens, 1600). If the coccygeal nerve is taken into account, 20 nerve roots make up the cauda equina which descends in the spinal

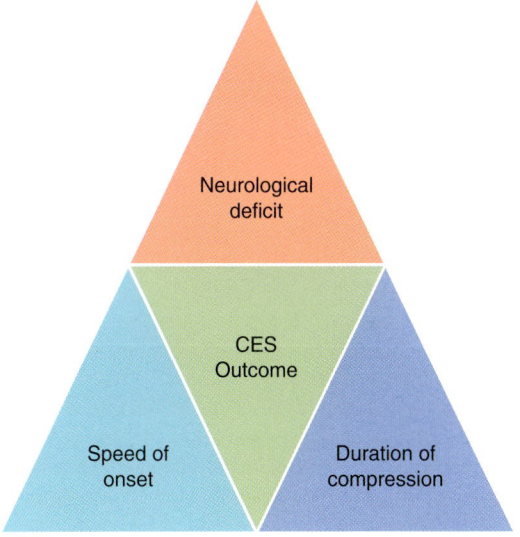

Fig. 5.2 Parameters determining outcome in CES.

canal from approximately the L1/2 level. The caudal nerve roots below the first lumbar root descend at an almost vertical angle to reach their corresponding foramina, gathered around the filum terminale (a continuation of the pia mater) within the spinal theca (Standring, 2009).

The first sacral nerve is the largest spinal nerve, thereafter decreasing in size quickly, with the coccygeal nerves being the smallest. According to Parke et al. (1981), the first three sacral nerves supply multifidus and lateral cutaneous branches to the skin and fascia over the sacrum and part of the gluteal region. The fourth and fifth sacral nerves, along with the posterior primary ramus of the coccygeal nerve, supply the skin and fascia around the coccyx. The pelvic splenic nerves to the pelvic viscera are composed of parasympathetic fibres and travel in the ventral rami of the second, third and fourth sacral spinal nerves. They then leave these nerves as they exit the anterior sacral foramina and pass to the presacral tissue. Some pass to the pelvic viscera alongside the pelvic sympathetic supply and supply the urogenital organs and distal aspect of the large intestine. Others pass directly into the retroperitoneal tissue and into the mesentery of the sigmoid and descending colon (Standring, 2009). The pudendal nerve supplies the perineum and arises from the second, third and fourth sacral nerves, with its terminal branches including the dorsal nerve of the penis or clitoris (Brash & Jamieson, 1937). The anal and bulbocavernosus reflexes depend on intact sacral arcs. The anal reflex can be seen with a visible contraction on perianal pin prick. Unfortunately, these reflexes are not reliable in relation to either diagnosis or prognosis (Grundy & Swain, 1996).

Cauda equina compression

The precise pathophysiology of CES is unknown but occurs as a result of direct compression of the lumbo-sacral nerve roots distal to the conus medialis. The most common cause of CES is compression arising from a large central lumbar disc herniation at the L4/5 or L5/S1 level (Mukherjee et al., 2013); however, CES can also be caused by compression via trauma, tumour, spinal canal stenosis, epidural haematoma or abscess or infection (Douraiswami et al., 2016). Patients with congenital narrowing of the spinal canal or acquired stenosis secondary to degenerative changes are consequently more at risk. It has been suggested that the proximal portion of the cauda equina is relatively hypovascular and in prime position for disc herniation causing compression (Parke et al., 1981). Blood supply alterations resulting from nerve root pressure may therefore be more important in this region of the cauda equina than elsewhere (Mukherjee et al., 2013). Additionally, the nerve roots comprising the cauda equina are particularly vulnerable to compression as there are no Schwann cells to produce a protective myelin sheath (Douraiswami et al., 2016)

Neural control of the bladder, bowel and sexual function

The neural control of bladder, bowel and sexual functions is governed by four systems:

- central sensory
- central motor
- peripheral sensory
- peripheral motor
  (Haldeman et al., 2002)

The autonomic nervous system maintains the internal environment by regulating visceral unconscious function throughout the body. It is composed of efferent and afferent neural tissue, which innervates the involuntary muscular system and glands. The efferent aspect of the autonomic system is composed of sympathetic and parasympathetic divisions. The afferent system is composed of visceral afferent fibres travelling in nerves that make up the sympathetic and parasympathetic divisions. Therefore, all viscera are innervated by sympathetic and parasympathetic afferent and efferent fibres (Table 5.1) (Young et al., 2015).

Sympathetic activity associated with the 'fight and flight' response enters the nervous system via the thoracolumbar spinal nerves, whereas parasympathetic activity related to 'rest and recuperation' or 'feed and breed', enters via the cranial and sacral roots. The parasympathetic division plays a huge role in both bladder and bowel continence, along with sexual arousal.

All parasympathetic activity arises from the brain stem or spinal cord. The sacral preganglionic parasympathetic neurones lay in or close to the spinal segments S2, 3 and 4 and may also be known as pelvic splenic nerves. The sacral parasympathetic nerves control elimination of waste and erection. Preganglionic fibres pass to the terminal ganglia of the colon, rectum, bladder, prostate and vaginal glands. The pelvic splenic efferent preganglionic cell bodies are in the lateral horn of the spinal cord at T12–L1 and their axons exit the vertebral column at S2–4 through the sacral foramen. These preganglionic neurons, unlike sympathetic neurones, synapse close to the organ of innervation. In general, the pelvic splenic nerves travel to one or more plexuses prior to reaching

TABLE 5.1 Autonomic nerve supply to the urogenital system (Young et al., 2015).

Organ	Sympathetic			Parasympathetic		
	Preganglionic	Postganglionic	Function	Preganglionic	Postganglionic	Function
Sex organs	T10–L1	Inferior hypogastric ganglia	Ejaculation	S2–4	Cavernous ganglia	Erection
Bladder	T12–L2	Hypogastric ganglia	Trigone muscle contraction	S2–4	Vesical ganglia	Contraction of detrusor muscle

BOX 5.1 The micturition cycle (Mtui et al., 2016).

- Anterior horn motor neurones to levator ani and muscles to pelvic floor are inhibited by micturition centre in pons
- Mucosal fibres of the pudendal nerve discharge impulses to the posterior grey horn of cord segments S2–4
- From the sacral cord, sensory neurones send impulses to the pontine micturition centre
- Sacral parasympathetic neurones serving the bladder are simultaneously stimulated
- Detrusor responds by contracting, expelling urine
- The rhabdosphincter contracts to expel urine from urethral canal
- Levator ani contracts to resume supportive role

the target organ or walls of the tissue they innervate. Mechanoreceptors in the bladder wall register fullness of the bladder. The fullness message is carried via the spino-thalamic tract to the thalamus and cortex. The sensation of need to micturate is triggered by mechanoreceptors in the trigone of the bladder. These visceral afferent messages travel with the sacral parasympathetic nerves to S2, 3 and 4 and ascend to the dorsal column (Young et al., 2015). Unconsciously, the parasympathetic nerve supply will cause peristalsis of the ureters and intestines, moving urine from the kidneys into the bladder. The parasympathetic supply will cause the urinary bladder wall detrusor muscle to contract. Simultaneously, the internal sphincter muscle between the bladder and the urethra will be stimulated to relax, resulting in voiding of bladder content (Box 5.1). Likewise, parasympathetic stimulation of the internal anal sphincter will relax this muscle to allow defecation.

Micturition centres are situated in the brain stem and cerebral cortex. Voluntary control for stopping and starting micturition is of cortical origin. One pontine micturition centre excites the sacral parasympathetic nerve supply and elicits contraction of the detrusor muscle. A second centre sends excitatory impulses to the lower motor neurones supplying the external urethral sphincters. Reflex bladder action is initiated via volume and tension visceral afferent receptors. Hence it is via a complex neural mechanism controlled by the spinopontospinal reflex that the external sphincter relaxes and the detrusor muscle contracts, thus emptying the bladder.

Problems such as CES disrupt this reflex action resulting in a neurogenic bladder.

There are two types of neurogenic bladder:

1. Reflex neurogenic bladder
   An upper motor lesion, resulting in a spastic bladder and leading to complete bladder voiding as a result of bilateral micturition centre lesions in the frontal lobe.

2. Non-reflex bladder
   A lower motor lesion resulting in a flaccid bladder. This is characterised by severe urinary retention and overflow incontinence due to damage to the spinal nerve roots in the cauda equina.

Unfortunately, bladder, bowel and sexual dysfunction, along with saddle anaesthesia, are all multi-factorial in their causes. In a retrospective review of 753 consecutive LBP patients in the UK, 28% of patients reported altered bladder and bowel function and 27% felt that their bladder and bowel control had changed with the onset of their LBP (Buchanan, 2013). Only one of these patients had a radiologically confirmed CES that was managed by emergency surgery. Acute urinary retention may result from any factor that obstructs, narrows or compresses the urethra which may subsequently prevent the passage of urine out of the body (Table 5.2).

The saddle area

Saddle anaesthesia is defined as reduced sensation affecting the saddle region, this being the area supplied by the S3, S4 and S5 nerves (Fig. 5.3; Standring, 2009).

During interviews and personal communication with CES sufferers, the extent of saddle numbness has been an interesting discussion point. One 32-year-old male CES sufferer described the saddle numbness as encompassing everything that anatomically touches the seat of a chair extending from the upper buttocks to upper thighs. These sufferers also described the difficulties that this lack of sensation brings with simple tasks such as stand-to-sit in relation to balance and control. Another male sufferer described his fear when, during the onset of his CES, he sat in the bath and could not feel any sensation of support beneath him. He described an unnerving sense of unsupported sitting with an associated fear of falling. This more extensive saddle region is illustrated in Fig. 5.4.

Bednar (2016) points out that urinary symptoms such as altered sensation, change in stream, loss of desire to void, hesitancy and straining to void are mostly S2 mediated, whereas perianal symptoms such as numbness or pain are mediated from the S2–4 segments.

Sexual dysfunction

Normal sexual functioning is defined as 'A complex biopsychosocial process that involves the coordinated actions of psychological, endocrine and vascular and neurological systems' (Shamloul and Ghanem, 2013). Similar to bladder and bowel dysfunction, sexual dysfunction is multi-factorial

TABLE 5.2 Potential red herrings causing bladder and or bowel dysfunction (Woods et al., 2015).

Benign prostatic hyperplasia (BPH)
Gynaecological problems such as ovarian cysts, uterine fibroids and organ prolapses (bladder, rectum or uterine) can cause acute urinary retention in women through external compression on the urethra
Gastrointestinal and retroperitoneal masses may cause urinary retention due to compression of the nearby bladder or urethra
Constipation, a side effect of common pain-relieving medication frequently prescribed in low back pain (LBP) can lead to bowel impaction, also causing external compression of the urethra
Urinary tract infections/cystitis and sexually transmitted diseases can cause local inflammation and urinary retention through temporarily narrowing the urethra in both men and women
Lyme disease, the varicella zoster virus and the herpes simplex virus have all been linked to cases of urinary retention
A single episode of pain in the pelvic region such as the onset of LBP is clinically known to cause urinary retention in some patients
Trauma to the sexual organs, for example, penile trauma, can lead to acute urinary retention. Postpartum complications and postoperative complications from pelvic surgery or pelvic trauma can also induce urinary retention. This may be due to damage to the pudendal nerve, which is located within the pelvis and supplies the bladder, bowel and sexual organs
Fowler's syndrome, a dysfunction of the urethral sphincter, may also cause acute urinary retention in young women
Psychogenic causes of acute urinary retention are also possible
Neurological conditions such as Parkinson's disease and multiple sclerosis
Cerebrovascular disease or a spinal cord injury may underpin upper motor neurone reasons for bladder dysfunction
Poorly controlled diabetes or radical pelvic surgery may cause damage to peripheral nerves supplying the bladder or bowel
Many medications used in the management of long-term conditions can also cause urinary retention

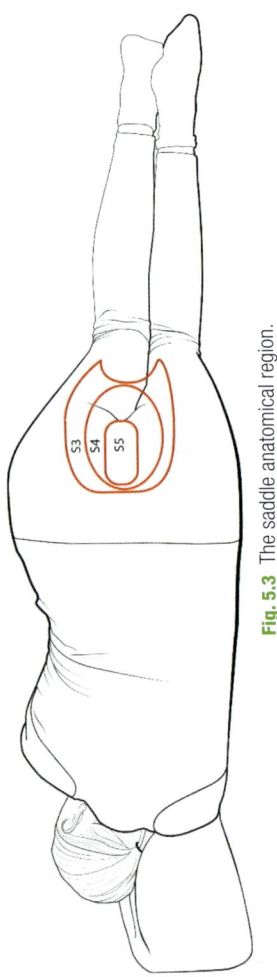

Fig. 5.3 The saddle anatomical region.

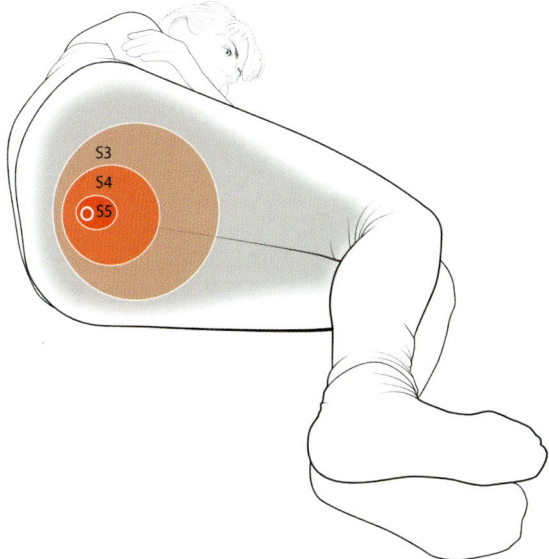

Fig. 5.4 The saddle region described by CES sufferers.

in its causes and is linked to a range of frequently seen medical conditions. Sexual dysfunction entails any problem that interferes with any of the normal phases of sexual activity, these being sexual interest or libido, sexual arousal, orgasm and resolution. Sexual dysfunction associated with CES can be complicated because of the diverse spectrum of problems reported.

Types of sexual dysfunction associated with CES (Korse et al., 2013):
- impotence
- decreased potency
- difficulties in obtaining orgasm

- less intense orgasm
- anorgasmy
- reduced or absent penile/vaginal sensation
- incontinence during intercourse
- dyspareunia
- absent bulbocavernosus reflex

As stated previously, there can be considerable therapist embarrassment in asking questions and patient embarrassment in responding to questions associated with these intimate problems which helped to stimulate us in developing the clinical cue card and patient credit card described later (Figs. 5.5 and 5.6).

Stages of CES

Clinicians commonly consider CES as either incomplete (CES-I) or complete (CES-R) (Gardner et al., 2011). More recently, there has been a move to include additional categories; a third category of CES early (CES-E) (Fairbank, 2014) more recently discussed as CES suspected (CES-S) (Todd & Dixon, 2016) and a fourth category of CES complete (CES-C) (Todd & Dickson, 2016) (Fig. 5.7).

Definitions of CES, differential diagnosis and Red Flags

Surprisingly, despite the vast body of literature, one of the fundamental challenges associated with CES is the lack of a precise definition of the condition. It is clear (Greenhalgh et al., 2018) that:

...there is no pattern to the development of CES signs and symptoms.

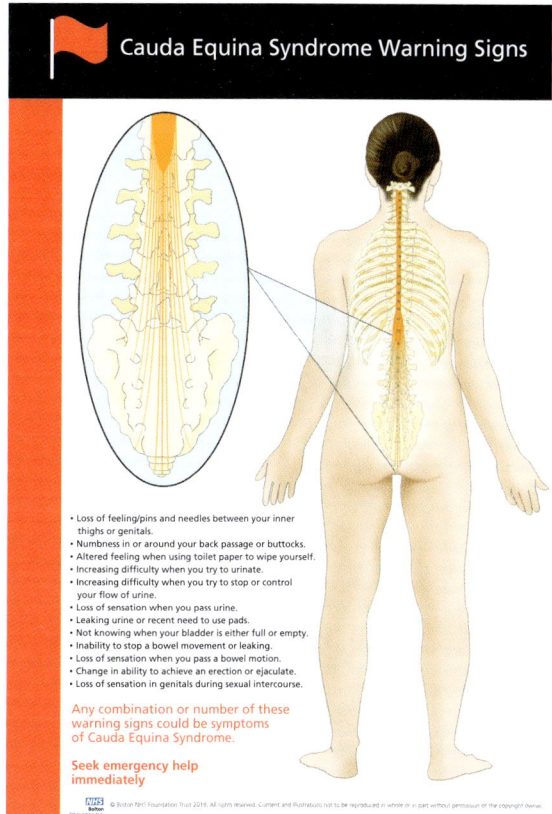

Cauda Equina Syndrome Warning Signs

- Loss of feeling/pins and needles between your inner thighs or genitals.
- Numbness in or around your back passage or buttocks.
- Altered feeling when using toilet paper to wipe yourself.
- Increasing difficulty when you try to urinate.
- Increasing difficulty when you try to stop or control your flow of urine.
- Loss of sensation when you pass urine.
- Leaking urine or recent need to use pads.
- Not knowing when your bladder is either full or empty.
- Inability to stop a bowel movement or leaking.
- Loss of sensation when you pass a bowel motion.
- Change in ability to achieve an erection or ejaculate.
- Loss of sensation in genitals during sexual intercourse.

Any combination or number of these warning signs could be symptoms of Cauda Equina Syndrome.

Seek emergency help immediately

© Bolton NHS Foundation Trust 2016. All rights reserved. Content and illustrations not to be reproduced in whole or in part without permission of the copyright owner.

Fig. 5.5 Clinician's CES cue card.

and that there is a vast range of potential signs and symptoms for clinicians to be aware of. This myriad of signs and symptoms highlights the complexity of trying to identify at-risk or potential CES patients early in the development

- Loss of feeling/pins and needles between your inner thighs or genitals
- Numbness in or around your back passage or buttocks
- Altered feeling when using toilet paper to wipe yourself
- Increasing difficulty when you try to urinate
- Increasing difficulty when you try to stop or control your flow of urine
- Loss of sensation when you pass urine
- Leaking urine or recent need to use pads
- Not knowing when your bladder is either full or empty
- Inability to stop a bowel movement or leaking
- Loss of sensation when you pass a bowel motion
- Change in ability to achieve an erection or ejaculate
- Loss of sensation in genitals during sexual intercourse

Any combination seek help immediately

Fig. 5.6 Patient's CES credit card.

CESS Suspected	• Bilateral radicular pain • (progressing unilateral)
CESI Incomplete	• Urinary difficulties of neurogenic origin • Altered urinary sensation • Loss of desire to void • Poor urinary stream • Need to strain to micturate
CESR Retention	• Painless urinary retention and overflow incontinence
CESC Complete	• Objective loss of CE function • Absent perineal sensation • Patulous anus (spread open) • Paralysed insensate bladder and bowel

Fig. 5.7 Four stages of CES (Todd & Dickson, 2016).

of what can be a very rapidly developing condition. However, knowing that there is 'no pattern' to look for is actually quite helpful clinically as most clinicians use a hypothetico-deductive reasoning approach where pattern recognition is central to successful diagnosis. The sensitivity and specificity for clinical examination of CES is low; therefore, most patients with clinical concern of CES do not actually have CES, and even clinical diagnosis made by neurosurgeons has a 43% false positive rate (Bell et al., 2007). Deyo et al., 1992 state that urinary retention has a sensitivity of 90%. In patients without urinary retention, the probability of CES is approximately 1 in 10,000. Fraser et al. (2009) confirm that there is a lack of a precise definition in their review of 105 papers. They highlighted numerous challenges and significant inconsistencies surrounding the aetiology and clinical presentation of CES and reported that there were 17 different definitions of CES. They went on to propose a new definition of CES based on a content analysis and synthesis of the numerous definitions that they had identified:

> *For a diagnosis of CES, one or more of the following must be present:*
>
> 1. *bladder and/or bowel dysfunction,*
> 2. *reduced sensation in the saddle area, and*
> 3. *sexual dysfunction, with possible neurologic deficit in the lower limb (motor/sensory loss, reflex change).*

Delitto et al. (2012) in the American Physical Therapy Association's *Low Back Pain: Clinical Practice Guidelines* report the following:

- urine retention: 0.90 sensitivity, 0.95 specificity, 18.0+ likelihood ratio (LR) (95% confidence interval [CI]), 0.11–LR (95% CI)
- saddle anaesthesia: 0.75 sensitivity
- sensory or motor deficits in the feet (L4, L5, S1 areas): 0.80 sensitivity

In 2015 the British Association of Spinal Surgeons (BASS) published their helpful standards of care for suspected and confirmed compressive CES in 2015 (Germon et al., 2015). In these standards they define CES as:

> *A patient presenting with acute (de novo or as an exacerbation of pre-existing symptoms) back pain and/or leg pain with a suggestion of a disturbance of their bladder or bowel function and/or saddle sensory disturbance should be suspected of having a CES.*

BASS (Germon et al., 2015) also highlight the low sensitivity and specificity for clinical examination of CES. In relation to suspected cases of CES they go on to say:

Most of these patients will not have critical compression of the cauda equina. However, in the absence of reliably predictive symptoms and signs, there should be a low threshold for investigation with an emergency scan. The reasons for not requesting a scan should be clearly documented.

CES is a clinical diagnosis confirmed by MRI. Although conducted commonly in clinical practice, the individual sensitivities of the following tests are relatively poor. This has in part been attributed to observer unfamiliarity with the clinical examination rather than the test itself (Bell et al., 2007; Fairbank et al., 2011). Suggested special objective tests and potentially worrying findings are as follows:

- perianal sensation reduced to light touch and/or pin prick
- loss or diminution of the bulbocavernosus reflex (reflex contraction of the anal sphincter caused by stimulation of the glans, penis or clitoris) as the reflex is mediated through the sacral roots which anatomically lie close to the L1 vertebra (Lavy et al., 2009)
- reduced sphincter tone on digital rectal examination (DRE)

DRE is just one aspect of the overall clinical examination but it generates a disproportionately large amount of discussion, probably due to the invasive and intimate nature of the examination. The accuracy of DRE is limited (Sherlock et al., 2015); however, it is a well-documented and essential examination procedure identified in multiple standards of care relating to CES (Germon et al., 2015; Todd & Dickson, 2016). A link between alteration in anal tone and subsequent spinal pathology has been identified in the latter part of the 20th century (Kostuik et al., 1986), and a strong correlation between anal sphincter tone, saddle paraesthesia and poor outcome has also been demonstrated (Kennedy et al., 1999). However, anal tone may be maintained in the presence of early CES—the optimum time for spinal surgery! As demonstrated by Sherlock et al. (2015), controversy surrounds the validity and reproducibility of the DRE technique itself. They constructed a model anus using a sphygmomanometer cuff; the cuff could be inflated to mimic normal or abnormal anal tone. Seventy-five doctors from a variety of specialities and 30 healthcare practitioners undertook DRE assessments. Although training on DRE was variable amongst the doctors, despite their medical experience, both groups had a mean accuracy of 64%. There was no correlation between experience of DRE and an individual's ability to perform the test. Sherlock et al. (2015) argue that the study demonstrates that previous experience and training does not enhance accuracy of DRE and suggest caution in interpreting this test in isolation. Recently, Angus et al. (2018) confirmed the limited clinical utility of DRE in a retrospective study of 309 patients presenting to an emergency department with suspected CES. The test with the lowest predictive value for CES was anal tone. Almost half of the non-compression group had reduced anal tone, with none of the compression group having any decrements in their anal tone whatsoever. Therefore, DRE findings must be interpreted with caution and considered in the context of the overall clinical picture, including the squeeze test, saddle sensation testing to light touch and pin prick and more importantly subjective symptoms. It is imperative that DRE findings alone are not used to ration onward investigation and referral. Interestingly, Angus et al. (2018) also identified no differences in light touch sensation and pin prick between compression and non-compression groups.

Todd & Dickson (2016) suggest five characteristic features of CES:

- bilateral neurogenic sciatica
- reduced perineal sensation
- altered bladder function ultimately to painless urinary retention
- loss of anal tone
- sexual dysfunction

Verhagen et al. (2016) reviewed the Red Flags presented in international guidelines on LBP and found 9 Red Fags that were recommended in relation to CES. Two Red Flags were frequently mentioned in numerous guidelines—'saddle anaesthesia (perineal numbness)', and '(sudden onset of) bladder dysfunction':

- saddle anaesthesia/perineal numbness
  Canada, Europe, Finland, France, Italy, New Zealand, United States
- (sudden onset) bladder dysfunction (e.g. urinary retention, overflow incontinence)
  Canada, Europe, Finland, France, Italy, New Zealand, United States
- sphincter disturbance/reduced tonus
  Canada, Europe, Finland, France, Italy, New Zealand
- progressive weakness in lower limbs/lower motor neuron weakness
  Europe, Finland, United States
- (wide) spread sensory deficit (in lower limbs)
  Italy, New Zealand
- gait disturbance/abnormality
  Europe, New Zealand
- faecal incontinence
  Canada, New Zealand
- pain (radiating) in both legs
  Canada, Italy
- sciatica
  France

Verhagen et al. (2016) concluded that there was a lack of consensus between guidelines on which Red Flags to endorse and that the evidence for the accuracy of any of the recommended Red Flags was lacking. Their aim was to facilitate early onward referral to specialist teams to avoid life-changing outcomes caused by delayed diagnosis.

More recently in 2018, the Medical Protection Society (MPS) was influential in the revision of the National Institute for Health and Care Excellence (NICE) Clinical Knowledge Summaries for Red Flags for cauda equina syndrome. The MPS maintains that formerly, Red Flag thresholds to refer on for urgent investigations were too high. They felt more explicit Red Flags were essential to facilitate early diagnosis and recommend the following Red Flags as potential triggers for onward referral:

- bilateral sciatica
- severe or progressive bilateral neurological deficit of the legs, such as major motor weakness with knee extension, ankle eversion or foot dorsiflexion
- difficulty initiating micturition or impaired sensation of urine flow (if untreated, this may lead to irreversible urinary retention with overflow urinary incontinence)
- loss of sensation of rectal fullness (if untreated, this may lead to irreversible faecal incontinence)
- perianal, perineal or genital sensory loss (saddle anaesthesia or paraesthesia)
- laxity of the anal sphincter tone

(MPS, 2018)

It is vital to realise that not all symptoms or signs will be present in any individual patient. The evidence presented in this section clearly shows there is no individual symptom, sign or combination that reliably diagnoses or excludes CES. Only by careful history-taking and relevant clinical examination can CES be diagnosed early and treated appropriately to avoid life-long disability. It is recognised that more accurate clinical diagnosis can be made late in the disease process when irreversible damage has often occurred (Todd & Dickson, 2016). However, the challenge, particularly in a first contact or primary care setting, is to make this critical diagnosis early when symptoms, especially those related to parasympathetic activity, can be more subtle and vague. We have previously reported how important it is that clinicians use a language and communication style that patients can understand (Greenhalgh et al., 2015). In addition, we have also highlighted that clinicians must frame the importance of questions related to serious pathology or else it is very easy for these key questions to come across as abstract and irrelevant, especially in the context of severe pain. To assist in consultations we have produced a cue card (Fig. 5.5), for clinicians to use in consultations which helps alleviate potential therapist embarrassment in asking questions and patient embarrassment in responding to questions, and a credit card (Fig. 5.6) reflecting the same information for patients to take away with them (Greenhalgh et al., 2016). This card has been translated into 28 languages (Table 5.3), and is available from Dynamic Health, Cambridgeshire Community Services' website: http://www.eoemskservice.nhs.uk/ or MACP website: https://macpweb.org/home/

Investigation (magnetic resonance imaging)

CES requires a clinical diagnosis confirmed by magnetic resonance imaging (MRI) to be accepted as a true diagnosis. An MRI is the gold standard investigation for this

TABLE 5.3 Listing CES patient credit card languages.

Arabic	Latvian
Bengali	Lithuanian
Cantonese	Mandarin
Czech	Polish
Dari	Portuguese
Farsi	Punjabi
French	Romanian
German	Russian
Greek	Slovak
Gujarati	Somali
Hindi	Spanish
Hungarian	Turkish
Italian	Urdu
Kurdish	Welsh

condition (Patel et al., 2016), as it effectively shows soft tissues including intervertebral discs, ligamentum flavum, dural sac and nerve roots (Mukherjee et al., 2013). Fairbank (2014) states the cause and level of the spinal pathology in CES can only be established with an MRI scan. As a consequence of the complexities of early CES symptoms, the high incidence of issues that contribute to symptoms that masquerade as CES and the dire consequence of late diagnosis, there is a justifiably high rate of negative CES compression found on MRI. Rates of MRI confirmed CES compression range from just 14% up to 33% (Todd & Dickson, 2016). However, clinicians should retain a low threshold for MRI where there are any relevant symptoms or signs; this will inevitably lead to a high number of MRI requests (in particular urgent/emergency MRIs) but this can be justified if it prevents or reduces the severe neurological morbidity that is associated with CES (Todd & Dickson, 2016). Germon et al. (2015)

concur that a large proportion of those scanned for symptoms suggestive of CES will not have critical compression. However, for a timely diagnosis of true CES to be made, a relatively low threshold to image must be adopted.

Fairbank (2014) suggests that the following symptoms of CES should prompt immediate MRI:

- bilateral sciatica
- bilateral paraesthesia
- bilateral motor deficit
- perineal pain
- perineal paraesthesia
- altered bladder/anal function
- bladder dysfunction

However, it must be noted that not all of these symptoms need to be present for a diagnosis of CES to be suspected and MRI organised.

Germon et al. (2015) provide helpful scenarios relating to the MRI outcome:

Cauda equina compression confirmed. This should precipitate an urgent referral to the appropriate surgical service.

Cauda equina compression excluded but a potential structural explanation of pain identified. This should precipitate appropriate advice which may include referral to the appropriate surgical service.

Non-compressive pathology may be identified (for example, demyelination). This should precipitate referral to the appropriate service.

No explanation of the patient's symptoms may be apparent in which case it is probably appropriate to refer back to the GP.

Domen et al. (2009) retrospectively studied 58 consecutive cases of suspected CES presenting to an emergency department. In the absence of strong predictive clinical characteristics for patients with CES, they recommend urgent MRI for every patient in the context of new onset urinary symptoms with an underlying LBP or sciatica. They go on to say that, although unnecessary MRIs will be carried out using this principle, they feel the numbers are still negligible in the context of potential permanent sphincter disruption and life-changing outcomes. Hassan et al. (2018) describe the poor availability of MRI scanning out-of-hours in general hospital settings which confounds the situation. These authors suggest a national policy for MRI scanning availability 24/7 at all hospitals to investigate suspected CES cases in a timely manner and avoid unnecessary referrals to overworked specialist spinal centres.

Identification of CES can, without a doubt, be challenging. Clinicians should retain a low threshold for suspicion and referral for further investigation, with MRI as the gold standard investigation. Emergency action is required to avoid permanent damage which can have devastating and life-changing consequences for patients and result in high-cost negligence claims, which we go on to discuss in the next chapter.

References

Angus M, Hamad O, Siddique I, Yasin N, Mc Creary R. *Can We Accurately Predict the Likelihood of Cauda Equina Syndrome in the Emergency Department*. Leeds: Poster BritSpine; 2018.

Bednar D. Cauda equina syndrome from lumbar disc herniation. *CMAJ.* 2016;188(4):284.

Bell DA, Collie D, Statham PF. Cauda equina syndrome: what is the correlation between clinical assessment and MRI scanning? *Br J Neurosurg.* 2007;21:201–203.

Brash J, Jamieson E, eds. *Cunninghams Textbook of Anatomy.* 7th ed. Oxford Medical Publications; 1937.

Buchanan E. How commonly do patients self-report subjective symptoms of cauda equina syndrome when asked on a screening form in a musculoskeletal triage service. *CSP Congress.* 2013.

Cyriax J. Cauda equina syndrome. *BMJ.* 1960;1:279.

Delitto A, George SZ, van Dillen L, et al. Low back pain: clinical practice guidelines linked to the International Classification of Functioning, Disability, and Health from the Orthopaedic Section of the American Physical Therapy Association. *J Orthop Sports Phys Ther.* 2012;42(4):A1–A57.

Deyo RA, Rainville J, Kent DL. What can the history and physical examination tell us about low back pain? *JAMA.* 1992;268(6):760–765.

Domen P, Hofman A, van Santbrink H, Weber W. Predictive value of clinical characteristics in patients with suspected cauda equina syndrome. *Eur J Neurol.* 2009;16:416–419.

Douraiswami B, Muthuswamy K, Naidu D, Thanigai S, Anand V. Indeterminate cauda equina syndrome: a case report. *J Clin Orthop Trauma.* 2016;1(7):50–54.

Du Laurens A. Historia anatomica humani corporis p. 153. https://books.google.co.uk/books?id=uFSEpz9vWNMC&pg=PP4&redir_esc=y#v=onepage&q=cauda%20equina&f=false; 1600.

Fairbank J, Hashimoto R, Dailey A, Patel AA, Dettori JR. Does patient history and physical examination predict MRI proven cauda equina syndrome? *Evid Based Spine Care J.* 2011;2:27–33.

Fairbank J. Cauda equina syndrome – risk management. *J Trauma and Orthop.* 2014;2(3):49–50.

Fraser S, Roberts L, Murphy E. Cauda equina syndrome: a literature review of its definition and clinical presentation. *Arch Phys Med Rehabil.* 2009;11:1964–1968.

Gardner A, Gardner E, Morley T. Cauda equina syndrome: a review of the current clinical and medico-legal position. *Eur Spine J.* 2011;20:690–697.

Germon T, Ahuja J, Casey A, et al. British association of spinal surgeons: standards of care for suspected and confirmed compressive CES. *Spine J.* 2015;15(2015):2S–4S.

Greenhalgh S, Truman C, Webster V, Selfe J. An investigation into the patient experience of cauda equina syndrome (CES). *Physiother Pract Res.* 2015;36:23–31.

Greenhalgh S, Truman C, Webster V, Selfe J. Development of a toolkit to manage cauda equina syndrome (CES). *Prim Health Care Res Dev*. 2016;17(6):559–567.

Greenhalgh S, Finucane L, Mercer C, Selfe J. Assessment and management of cauda equina syndrome. *Musculoskelet Sci Pract*. 2018;37:69–74.

Grieve GP. *Mobilisation of the Spine*. 3rd ed. Edinburgh: Churchill Livingstone; 1979.

Grundy D, Swain A. *ABC of Spinal Cord Injury*. 3rd ed. BMJ Publishing Group; 1996.

Haldeman S, Kirkaldy-Willis W, Bernards T. *An Atlas of Back Pain*. The Parthenon Publishing Group; 2002.

Hassan M, Razak A, Hassan S, Choudhari K, Spink G. Time to implement a national referral pathway for suspected cauda equina syndrome: review and outcome of 250 referrals. *Br J Neurosurg*. 2018;32(3):264–268.

Kennedy J, Soffe K, McGrath A, et al. Predictors of outcome in cauda equina syndrome. *Eur Spine J*. 1999;8:317–322.

Korse N, Jacobs W, Elzevier H, Vleggeert- Lankamp C. Complaints of micturition, defecation and sexual function in cauda equina syndrome due to lumbar disk herniation: a systematic review. *Eur Spine J*. 2013;22:1019–1029.

Kostuik J, Harrington I, Alexander D, et al. Cauda equina syndrome and lumbar disk herniation. *J Bone Joint Surg Am*. 1986;68A:386–391.

Lavy C, James A, Wilson-MacDonald J, Fairbank J. Cauda equina syndrome. *BMJ*. 2009;338:b936.

Maitland GD. *Vertebral Manipulation*. 4th ed. London: Butterworths; 1977.

McKenzie RA. *The Lumbar Spine Mechanical Diagnosis and Therapy*. Waikanae: Spinal Publications; 1981.

Medical Protection Society (MPS). 2018. Available online at: https://www.medicalprotection.org/uk/.

Mennell J. *The Science and Art of Manipulation: The Spinal Column*. 1st ed. London: J & A Churchill Ltd; 1952.

Mtui E, Gruener G, Dockerty P. *Clinical Neuroanatomy and Neuroscience*. Elsevier; 2016.

Mukherjee S, Thakur B, Crocker M. Cauda equina syndrome: a clinical review for the frontline clinician. *Br J Hosp Med*. 2013;74(8):460–464.

Parke WW, Gammell K, Rothman RH. Arterial vascularization of the cauda equina. *J Bone Joint Surg Am*. 1981;63:53–62.

Patel ND, Broderick DF, Burns J, et al. ACR appropriateness criteria low back pain. *J Am Coll Radiol*. 2016;13(9):1069–1078.

Price K. Towards a history of medical negligence. *Lancet*. 2010;375:192–193.

Shamloul R, Ghanem H. Erectile Dysfunction. *Lancet*. 2013;381:153–165.

Sherlock K, Turner W, Elsayed S, et al. The evaluation of digital rectal examination for assessment of anal tone in suspected cauda equina syndrome. *Spine*. 2015;40(15):1213–1218.

Standring S. *Gray's Anatomy*. 40th ed. Churchill Livingstone; 2009.

Todd N. Causes and outcomes of cauda equina syndrome in medico-legal practice: a single neurosurgical experience of 40 consecutive cases. *Br J Neurosurg*. 2011;25(4):503–508.

Todd N, Dickson D. Standards of care in cauda equina syndrome. *Br J Neurosurg*. 2016;30(5):518–522.

Verhagen AP, Downie A, Popal N, Maher C, Koes BW. Red Flags presented in current low back pain guidelines: a review. *Eur Spine J*. 2016;25:2788–2808.

Woods E, Greenhalgh S, Selfe J. Cauda equina syndrome and the challenge of diagnosis for physiotherapists: a review. *Physiother Pract Res*. 2015;36:81–86.

Young PA, Young PH, Tolbert D. *Basic Clinical Neurosience*. 3rd ed. Wolters Kluwer; 2015.

CHAPTER 6

Cauda Equina Syndrome: Consequences and Care

Although many standards of care for the management of cauda equina syndrome (CES) have been put forward, none have been unanimously accepted (Todd & Dickenson, 2016). In 2015, The British Association of Spinal Surgeons (BASS) produced standards of care for CES based on a consensus of members of the society (Germon et al., 2015). These particular standards were developed in response to BASS members' perceptions that some patients may be suffering from CES as a consequence of delayed diagnosis and surgery. This perception is one shared by many authors and it is also known that there is an association between delayed diagnosis and the risk of litigation (Mukherjee et al., 2013). Despite these standards of care, the optimal advice surrounding diagnosis and management of CES still remains under debate (Todd & Dickenson, 2016). As discussed in the previous chapter, diagnosis at an early stage in the disease process is challenging, compounding the risk of delayed diagnosis and resulting in life-changing consequences.

CES surgery in the 20th century

Between André du Lauren's first description of the cauda equina in 1600 and the early 20th century, cauda equina compression was recognised as a clinical problem. However, it was mostly presumed that the compression was caused by carcinoma of the vertebra. Early in the 20th century there was a shift in anatomical and clinical understanding and surgical papers from this period started reporting on cases of cauda equina compression due to intervertebral disc herniation rather than carcinoma. Elsberg (1916) is the earliest reference appearing in some of the pioneering surgical papers that describes a chondroma of the vertebra causing compression of the cauda equina. It is, however, Dandy (1929) who presented the first paper, a case report, that described cauda equina compression as being specifically attributable to disc herniation. In this paper he comments that:

> ...a review of the literature has failed to disclose other cases of their kind.

He goes on to describe two cases of cauda equina compression caused by disc herniations which were treated surgically:

> The lesion is a completely detached fragment of cartilage from an intervertebral (lumbar) disk and is surrounded by serum. It bulges dorsally into the spinal canal as a tumor, and by compressing the roots of the cauda equina causes motor and sensory paralysis...

Mixter and Barr, who presented a case history of cauda equina compression due to disc herniation in their widely quoted seminal 1934 paper on *Rupture of the intervertebral disc with involvement of the spinal canal*, are often incorrectly credited with being the first authors to coin the term 'cauda equina syndrome' (Mixter and Barr, 1934). It is unknown who actually coined the term. The first paper that specifically uses the term 'cauda equina compression syndrome' in the title appears to have been published by French and Payne in 1944 (French and Payne, 1944). In this paper, they presented a series of eight case histories of CES caused by vertebral disc herniation that were treated with surgical decompression. In their discussion, they presented a guide to clinicians which is still remarkably relevant over 70 years later:

> *These patients may serve, also, to illustrate a possible danger in delaying operation for displaced intervertebral disk either because of faulty diagnosis or election. Nearly all had evidence of long preexisting discogenic disease yet the diagnosis was not made until all had evidence of extensive cauda equina compression. They were, thereby, subjected to extensively prolonged hospitalization and convalescence, and to the real possibility of crippling neurologic residuum. In view of the fact that many of these patients had minimal complaints prior to the acute episode culminating in cauda equina compression, it seems possible that any patient with discogenic disease might potentially suffer a similar fate.*

Howard Black, reporting on a series of 11 case histories of CES just a few years later in 1948, echoes this sentiment when he states (Black, 1948):

> *Prompt surgical intervention is essential to satisfactory recovery. An instance is cited in which there was a prolonged period between onset of involvement of the cauda equina and operation. In this case almost no recovery has occurred, in contrast to reasonably good recoveries made by patients operated on soon after onset of compression of the cauda equina.*

CES surgery in the 21st century

The current recommendation from the BASS is unequivocal (Germon et al., 2015):

> *Nothing is to be gained by delaying surgery and potentially much to be lost. Decompressive surgery should be undertaken at the earliest opportunity…*

Clear guidance relating to the optimum timing for surgery has not always been readily available, particularly in the early 21st century. Despite some of the earlier surgical reports advocating early surgery, the optimal timing has, over the years, been controversial because of the lack of prospective randomised trials, and because, in several of the retrospective studies published, there have been inadequately defined time intervals between symptoms and surgery or mixed-patient cohorts including both incomplete CES (CES-I) and retention CES (CES-R), which have precluded robust conclusions (Mukherjee et al., 2013).

> *Only 4–7% of clinically suspected cases of CES require emergency surgery.*
>
> **Todd & Dickson, 2016**

Ahn et al. (2000) conducted a meta-analysis to determine correlation between timing of decompressive surgery and clinical outcome. They identified a significant advantage to surgery within 48 hours of the onset of CES as opposed to more than 48 hours. In 2002, Gleave & Macfarlane produced what was then seen as a pivotal paper (Gleave and Macfarlane, 2002). They presented CES in two stages—incomplete and complete. At that time, they suggested that patients suffering incomplete CES (i.e. not in retention) should be considered for emergency surgery. This is still in line with current BASS recommendations (Germon et al., 2015). This population were deemed to have a good surgical prognosis. However, those suffering from complete CES (i.e. with retention) of more than 48 hours were different. Contrary to current BASS recommendations (Germon et al., 2015), these patients were considered not to be adversely affected by delaying surgery as their neurological prognostic status was already considered to be poor (Gleave & Macfarlane, 2002). A safe window of 48 hours was proposed and subsequently widely accepted. Nevertheless, these patients would still be considered for emergency surgery but at the next practical opportunity. More recently, authors such as Chau et al. (2014) refute the proposition of a safe time to delay surgery. Their systematic clinical review identifies no strong evidence to support a safe delay window of surgery of 48 hours.

Fairbank (2014) cites the Society of British Neurological Surgeons' guidance which concludes that surgery should be immediate, highlighting the simple yet insightful quote:

> Nothing is to be gained by delaying surgery and potentially much to be lost.

Sun et al. (2014) present a large-scale and detailed analysis of the patterns of development of CES symptoms. They propose that patients with early signs of CES (CES-E) should be considered for surgery before CES signs and symptoms develop, specifically when symptoms are progressing, especially when progression from unilateral to bilateral leg pain is occurring. Interestingly, this early CES-E stage strongly reflects the approach suggested by

Cyriax (1960) some years earlier. Despite controversy around the optimum timing of surgical intervention, this surgical decision has always been for those expert clinicians in the surgical team. The task of the frontline clinician is, and has always been, to investigate and/or refer on suspected cases immediately (Mukherjee et al., 2013) (see later section on Clinical Pathways).

The decision to refer in the early stages must be carefully thought through based on the patient's individual presentation rather than on a set of rules. The resounding message from experts in the field of CES is that early, emergency surgery for these CES patients is advocated.

Dhatt et al. (2011) highlight an important perspective. Their retrospective study carried out in India was unusual in that they analysed the outcome of 50 patients who all presented to the surgical team late in the CES disease process (mean delay 12.2 days) and underwent decompression surgery soon after late presentation. They highlight that recovery time post-decompression for CES is much slower than that seen in more common intervertebral disc surgery. However, their findings illustrate that even late decompression may still provide some favourable outcomes, although neurological function, especially autonomic function, takes much longer in this population of patients, if indeed recovery is achieved at all. Tamburrelli et al. (2014) confirm the need for long-term follow-up to establish ultimate outcome in these patients. They carried out an observational study of eight male patients who presented to their surgical centre between 2007 and 2009. They confirmed the slow recovery times previously reported throughout literature. They observed that in this small study, one case that presented with significant neurological impairment had a poor outcome. However, seven patients monitored over several years improved significantly. Although the management of CES remains controversial, it remains clear that the timely opinion of the surgical team is of paramount importance no matter how long the CES symptoms have been present.

Surgical counselling

Germon et al. (2015) suggest that all patients undergoing surgery for CES should be counselled that the aim of surgery intervention is to preserve that function present at the time of surgery. It should be explained that there is some possibility of improvement but there is a small chance of worsening symptoms, including paralysis, loss of bladder and bowel control and significant sexual dysfunction, such as impotence.

Litigation

Physiotherapists need to decide in a limited timeframe whether the patient's problem is suitable for physiotherapy management (keep) or whether the patient needs to be referred to other medical personnel or sent for further investigation prior to the commencement of physiotherapy (refer). The physiotherapist has a professional duty of care and a legal responsibility to provide appropriate and timely care. In suspected CES, this duty of care is clearly to refer in a timely manner rather than to keep. Current World Confederation of Physical Therapy (WCPT) guidelines describe keep/refer decision-making as a core element of physiotherapy practice in the management of patients with potentially serious medical pathologies such as CES. However, there is huge variation in the way individual countries include reference to this element of physiotherapy practice within national guidelines (Lackenbauer et al., 2017). To help protect themselves from litigation, it is imperative that readers of this book practising outside the UK acquaint themselves with the relevant locally agreed standards of practice governing keep/refer decision-making in cases of potentially serious medical pathologies that are pertinent to their location.

In 2014, the Chartered Society of Physiotherapy (CSP) in the UK posted a 2-page document, *Learning from litigation,* online that presented key messages about CES (CSP, 2014). This document highlighted the change in the role of physiotherapists that has taken place over the past 20 years where it stated:

> *Physiotherapists see many patients with back pain, a large number of whom may come directly to see a physiotherapist without seeing a doctor first. As autonomous and accountable diagnostic practitioners, physiotherapists of all levels of experience need to be able to identify those patients who need urgent medical review and act accordingly.*

The paper goes onto describe how physiotherapists are now much more likely to be involved in cases of litigation for CES than they once were:

> *The basis for the claim is that the practitioner failed to: examine the patient properly; act on 'red flags' present, refer on or investigate with sufficient urgency. This does not just affect doctors and surgeons. Physiotherapists have been found to be clinically negligent for failing to act and/ or refer on when a patient presented with possible CES.*

More recently, the CSP, 2017 commissioned a clinical update and accompanying video both of which give good advice on how to manage patients with suspected

CES. The clinical update appears to be freely available at: http://www.csp.org.uk/frontline/article/clinical-update-cauda-equina-syndrome

It is also available to CSP members (if you are a member you will need to log in to view the video):

http://www.csp.org.uk/publications/learning-litigation-cauda-equina-syndrome-ces

The video is also available on line via Youtube at:

https://www.youtube.com/watch?v=8rRq5QqoK3o

CES is the number one 'spinal' patient safety issue for orthopaedic surgeons providing on-call and emergency care (Lavy et al., 2009). It is widely accepted that the rise in litigation is not due to an increasing incidence of clinical negligence, but rather 'the increasing tendency [of patients] to seek legal redress and the rising costs of such legal settlements' (Chacko, 2009). The current litigation situation compared to the past is three-pronged: health professionals, including physiotherapists, are being sued more often; when sued, they are more likely to lose; and when losing, the claims awarded against them are increasing in size. In the year ending 2004, the total cost of immediately paying all outstanding clinical negligence claims was £7.78 billion, which equates to approximately 13% of the UK National Health Service (NHS) budget. The average compensation awarded due to missed or delayed diagnosis of CES is £336,000 per case in the UK and $549,427 per case in the USA (Fairbank, 2014). The highest settlement for a single case of CES between 2003 and 2008 was £2,041,000 (Todd & Dickson, 2016). As patients become increasingly aware that health professionals are more likely to lose when sued for CES and that the courts are more likely to award larger settlements, the frequency with which lawsuits are pursued will almost certainly escalate (Chacko, 2009).

Modern medical negligence law can be distilled down to three fundamental factors (Price, 2010):

1. Confirming the patient was 'owed a legal duty of care' by the health practitioner, who is the 'defendant' in cases of medical negligence
2. Establishing that the defendant was in 'breach' of that duty of care in failing to reach the standard of care required by law
3. Proving that this breach of duty caused or contributed to the damage or injury to the patient. 'Reasonable practice' by a reasonable practitioner is used to establish what the standard of care is and if this had been breached and, consequently, if the breach was a causal factor in the outcome

Fairbank (2014) is clear:

> *If you think someone might have CES, even without signs, you should consider getting a scan and you MUST warn of the symptoms of deterioration and advise immediate re-attendance.*

If a patient has not developed any Red Flag symptoms at the time of the consultation, a medical negligence claim can still potentially be brought on the basis that the patient was not advised to report back if they did develop symptoms (Cauda Equina Syndrome Compensation Claim Solicitors, 2016). This issue around safety netting of the 'at risk' patient has helped provide the stimulus to develop the patient credit card (Fig. 5.6).

The following table presents the current advice to patients visiting the Cauda Equina Syndrome Compensation Claim Solicitors website who are considering launching a medicolegal claim (Box 6.1).

Finally, it is essential that a contemporaneous accurate record of the consultation and of the advice given appears in the patients notes as 'if it wasn't recorded, it didn't happen' (Fairbank, 2014). This is pertinent when considering the findings of Leerar et al. (2007), who reviewed the clinical charts of 160 patients with low back pain seen at six outpatient physical therapy clinics in the USA, noting the presence or absence of 11 Red Flags:

- age (50 and over)
- bladder dysfunction
- cancer history
- immune suppression
- rest/night pain
- trauma
- saddle anaesthesia
- lower extremity neurological deficit
- weight loss
- recent infection
- fever/chills

Documentation of Red Flags was comprehensive in some areas but lacking in others. The Red Flags that were most regularly documented were age over 50, bladder dysfunction, history of cancer, immune suppression, night pain, history of trauma, saddle anaesthesia and lower extremity neurological deficit. The Red Flags not regularly documented were weight loss, recent infection and fever/chills. In the context of CES, it is encouraging that the following percentages were recorded for the Red Flags of bladder dysfunction (100%), saddle anaesthesia (98.7%) and lower extremity neurological deficit (98.7%).

Clinical pathway

(In other words, what do you do when you have a patient in front of you that you suspect has CES)

BOX 6.1 What patients need to prove in order to establish medical negligence (Cauda Equina Syndrome Compensation Claim Solicitors, 2016).

If you believe that there has been a delay in diagnosing or treating your cauda equina syndrome, you will have to prove two elements in order to establish medical negligence:

- That failure to diagnose/suspect/warn of Red Flag symptoms would not be supported by a responsible body of medical opinion (in other words that there was breach of the duty of care owed to you)
- That the delay in diagnosing your cauda equina syndrome has led to a worse outcome for you (causation)

The first step in investigating a medical negligence claim on the basis of a delay in diagnosis or treating cauda equina syndrome is to obtain all of your medical records. These will then be sent to independent medical experts who will prepare opinions on the standard of care you received and whether any breach of duty has caused you to suffer further injury.

Many authors (Fairbank, 2014; Daniels et al., 2012; Strigenz, 2014) advocate the importance of cautioning patients at risk of CES of the signs and symptoms to be aware of and the timing of and precise action to take should these symptoms occur. Daniels et al. (2012) suggest that all patients suffering from back pain should be cautioned, whereas Fairbank (2014) stresses the importance of warning patients suspected of progressing to CES of the signs and symptoms to look out for and what immediate action to take:

You MUST warn of symptoms of deterioration and advise immediate re-attendance.

Fairbank, 2014

BOX 6.2 Sussex musculoskeletal (MSK) partnership standards of care (CES Pathway).

Documentation of cauda equina syndrome (CES)
No documentation = no evidence

The following signs and symptoms should be documented:
- Change in bladder control including ability to pass urine
- Change in bowel control including ability to open bowels
- Saddle anaesthesia
- Change in sexual function
  NB: Questioning should be framed to highlight the importance and seriousness of the condition, along with focusing the patient on sometimes subtle and vague early signs in a way that patients understand. It is crucial to use language that the patient understands. You may need to explore further questioning depending on the patient's response.

  If suspicious of CES document the following:
- Time and date you spoke to the patient
- Suspicious of CES and timescale of CES symptoms
- Document the action taken, e.g. referral to A&E, who you spoke to, and what time

  If patient at risk of developing CES document the following:
- Safety net (warn) the patient what to look out for
- Provide literature/card informing patient what signs and symptoms to look out for
- Clear advice of action they should take if they develop signs and symptoms and in what time frame to act

Strigenz (2014) concurs by suggesting that patients should be educated to enable them to become their own advocates.

Box 6.2 contains an example of standards of care embedded within a CES pathway currently used in the south of England.

The importance of your local CES pathway cannot be underestimated. For example, it is Friday and it is

4 pm. What are you going to do when the next patient who walks in is a suspected CES sufferer? Crucially, the pathway needs to facilitate appropriate imaging and surgical opinion on the same day whilst not encouraging unnecessary admission of those with negative CES, who will be in the majority. Physiotherapists can play an important role in bringing the patient and surgical team together in a timely manner, whilst avoiding unnecessary hospital admission. If surgical intervention is delayed, irreversible damage can occur to the bladder, bowel and sexual function with ongoing chronic pain. This is increasingly likely to lead to litigation. If CES is suspected, physiotherapists have a duty of care to refer and emergency magnetic resonance imaging (MRI) must be carried out on the same day to confirm or negate CES.

Nothing is to be gained by delaying surgery and potentially much to be lost.

Surgery should be carried out as soon as is practically possible.
Germon et al., 2015; Todd & Dickson, 2016

CASE

The following is a hypothetical case presenting in various ways to test your clinical decision-making. Our suggested management for the clinical conundrum is illustrated in red below each setting.

1. Jennifer is referred to you urgently with back pain. She has suffered from one episode of incontinence of urine 2 weeks ago but has had no other similar problems

since. Within the wider detailed subjective and objective examination, no other positive items on the CES cue card below are identified (Fig. 6.1).

Q: What will you do?

A: Safety Net

2. Jennifer has back and left leg pain to the knee and feels as if she is going to the toilet a little more frequently to pass urine. The pain in her leg is getting worse and is now radiating distally below the knee. Nothing else on the CES cue card is positive and there is no neurological deficit to find.

Q: What will you do?

A: Safety Net and MRI soon (this timescale must be agreed within pathway)

The important thing is to safety net. Ensure Jennifer is aware she needs to act immediately if things get worse

3. Jennifer has back and left leg pain to the ankle and has increased her dose of pregabalin as a result of her GP consultation. Since her medication has increased, Jennifer has had intermittent episodes of nocturnal incontinence. Neurological examination is unremarkable, sphincter tone and perianal sensation are normal.

Q: What will you do?

A: MRI immediately

(The change in bladder function is likely to be due to the medication but you can't take the risk)

4. Jennifer has now developed some numbness of the left side of the vagina.

Q: Now what will you do?

A: MRI immediately/refer onto emergency pathway

References

Ahn UM, Ahn NU, Buchowksi MS, Garrett ES, Sieber AN, Kostuik JP. Cauda equina syndrome secondary to lumbar disc herniation: a meta-analysis of surgical outcomes. *Spine*. 2000;25:1515–1522.

Black H. Massive herniation of the intervertebral disc producing compression of the cauda equina. *Calif Med*. 1948;69(4):271–274.

Cauda Equina Syndrome Compensation Claim Solicitors. 2016. http://www.cauda-equina.co.uk/can-i-make-claim/guide-to-a-cauda-equina-compensation-claim.

Chacko D. Medical liability litigation: an historical look at the causes for its growth in the United Kingdom. University of Oxford, Discussion Papers in Economic and Social History, Number 77. 2009.

Chartered Society of Physiotherapy. Learning from litigation: 1 - Cauda equina syndrome (CES). 2014. http://www.csp.org.uk/publications/learning-litigation-cauda-equina-syndrome-ces.

Chau A, Xu L, Pelzer N, Gragnaniello C. Timing of surgical intervention in cauda equina syndrome; a systematic review. *World Neurosurg*. 2014;81(3–4):640–650.

Cyriax J. Cauda equina syndrome. *BMJ*. 1960;1:279.

Dandy W. Loose cartilage from intervertebral disc simulating tumour of the spinal cord. *Arch Surg*. 1929;19(4):660–672.

Daniels E, Gordon Z, French K, Ahn U, Ahn N. Review of medicolegal cases for cauda equina syndrome; what factors lead to an adverse outcome for the provider? *Orthopaedics*. 2012;35(3):414–419.

Dhatt S, Tahasildar N, Tripathy S, Bhadur R, Dhillon M. Outcome of spinal decompression in cauda equina syndrome presenting late in developing countries: case series of 50 cases. *Eur Spine J*. 2011;20:2235–2239.

Elsberg CA. *Diagnosis and Treatment of Surgical Diseases of the Spinal Cord and Its Membranes*. Philadelphia: WB Saunders and Co; 1916.

Fairbank J. Cauda equina syndrome-risk management. *J Trauma Orthop*. 2014;2(3):49–50.

French J, Payne J. Cauda equina compression syndrome with herniated nucleus pulposus. *Ann Surg*. 1944;120(1):73–87.

Germon T, Ahuja S, Casey A, Rai A. British association of spinal surgeons standards of care for cauda equina syndrome. *Spine J*. 2015;15(3):S2–S4.

Gleave JRW, Macfarlane R. Cauda equina syndrome: what is the relationship between timing of surgery and outcome? *Br J Neurosurg*. 2002;16:325–328.

Lackenbauer W, Janssen J, Roddam H, Selfe J. Is keep/refer decision making an integral part of national guidelines for the physiotherapy profession within Europe? A review. *Physiotherapy*. 2017;103(4):352–360.

Lavy C, James A, Wilson-MacDonald J, Fairbank J. Cauda equina syndrome. *BMJ*. 2009;338:b936.

Leerar PJ, Boissonnault W, Domholdt E, Roddey T. Documentation of red flags by physical therapists for patients with low back pain. *J Man ManipTher*. 2007;15(1):42–49.

Mixter W, Barr J. Rupture of the intervertebral disc with involvement of the spinal canal. *N Engl J Med*. 1934;211:210–215.

Mukherjee S, Thakur B, Crocker M. Cauda equina syndrome; a clinical review for the frontline clinician. *Br J Hosp Med*. 2013;74(8):460–464.

Price K. Towards a history of medical negligence. *Lancet*. 2010;375:192–193.

Strigenz T. Cauda equina syndrome. *J Pain Palliat Care Pharmacother*. 2014;28:75–77.

Sun JC, Xu T, Chen KF, Qian W, Liu K, Shi JG, et al. Assessment of cauda equina syndrome progression pattern to improve diagnosis. *Spine*. 2014;39(7):596–602.

Tamburrelli F, Genitiempo M, Bochicchio M, Donisi L, Ratto C. Cauda equina syndrome: evaluation of the clinical outcome. *Eur Rev Med Pharmacol Sci*. 2014;18:1098–1105.

Todd NV, Dickenson RA. Standards of care in cauda equina syndrome. *Br J Neurosurg*. 2016;30(5):518–522.

CHAPTER 7

Metastatic Spinal Cord Compression (MSCC)

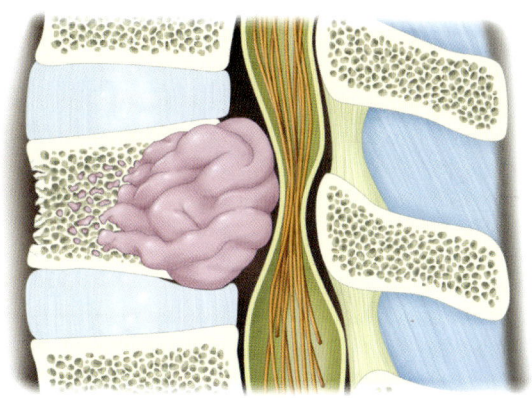

Metastatic spinal cord compression.

It is 4.00 pm on a Friday afternoon and your last patient of the week has just arrived for his first appointment. Mr Smith is 64 years old and complains of pain in his thoracic spine which radiates anteriorly around his chest. His legs feel odd and he reports that he has recently started to trip and stumble. He describes the pain as getting worse at night and during the last week he has slept upright in a chair as going to bed is too painful.

What are you going to do next?

It is of paramount importance to recognise metastatic spinal cord compression (MSCC) early to optimise patient outcomes. Primary care physiotherapists, first contact practitioners, physiotherapists, advanced practitioners, community nurses and GPs are perfectly placed to assist in early identification of MSCC.

However, it is well documented that diagnosis is commonly delayed. Tsukada et al. (2015) conducted a study to investigate factors that delay diagnosis. They identified that patients presenting with normal gait frequently suffered diagnostic delays. In addition, the number of days delayed was higher when weekends were included. It is essential to avoid delay in order that spinal stability and neurological function can be preserved. Once compression of the spinal cord occurs, it goes through a number of pathophysiological changes. Initially, the cord becomes oedematous and demyelination occurs, along with venous congestion. At this stage changes are reversible. If compression continues, the vascular injury and cord compression leads to permanent change (Robson, 2014; Kaplow & Iyere, 2016).

Background

In 2012, cancer was responsible for 1.26 million deaths in the 28 EU member states, with breast cancer alone causing 91,500 deaths (Ponti et al., 2017). Table 7.1 lists the top three cancers in the EU for males and females. A huge variation exists in the mortality rates from cancer across the member states of the EU, with cancer as the second most common cause of death in the UK. In England, survival with lung cancer remains very low, with 1-year survival below 45% and 5-year survival below

TABLE 7.1 The most common cancers in the European Union (European age standardised rate [E-ASR]).

Males	Females
Prostate cancer (E-ASR 110.8/100,000)	Breast cancer (E-ASR 108.8/100,000)
Lung cancer (E-ASR 66.3/100,000)	Colorectal cancer (E-ASR 36.1/100,000)
Colorectal cancer (E-ASR 59.0/100,000)	Lung cancer (E-ASR 26.1/100,000)

20% (Office for National Statistics, 2017). It is perhaps surprising that in the UK, 25% of cancers are diagnosed through Accident & Emergency (A&E) departments, and late diagnosis of cancer is related to older age as one-third of cancer diagnoses in the over 70s are made in A&E; late diagnosis results in lower survival rates in the first year (Ellis-Brookes et al., 2012).

Metastases are secondary malignant growths that develop at a distance away from a primary site of cancer. They form as cancer cells are able to break away from the primary cancer, travel through the blood or lymph system and form new tumours. The new metastatic tumour is the same type of cancer as the primary tumour. The spine is the most common site of metastases, occurring in 3%–5% of all patients with cancer, and can be one of the earliest sites affected (Brooks et al., 2014; Robson, 2014). Hartvigsen et al. (2018) identify that 97% of spinal tumours are metastatic in nature. Past history of cancer is the most useful Red Flag in relation to subsequent metastatic disease. However, the probability is only increased by 7% in primary care and 33% in an emergency setting (Hartvigsen et al., 2018).

In relation to MSCC, the true incidence is not known as most countries have no system to record the number of MSCC cases seen (Al Qurainy & Collis, 2016). Estimates of MSCC vary: Kwok et al. (2006) suggest progression to MSCC occurs in 5%–10% of cancer sufferers; there are approximately 4000 recorded cases of MSCC in England & Wales per annum (National Institute for Health and Care Excellence (NICE), 2008); Robson (2014) estimated the incidence to be 15% of patients with advanced cancer; and Al-Qurainy & Collis (2016) suggested that between 5 and 10 terminal cancer patients in every 200 develop MSCC within the last 2 years of life.

The most common primary cancers to metastasise to the spine are:

• lung
• breast
• prostate

These three cancers make up approximately 50% of MSCC tumours (Coleman & Holen, 2014).

Along with the lymph nodes, liver and lungs, the spinal cord is one of the most likely sites to be affected by metastases (Kaplow & Iyere, 2016). Back pain is the most common initial symptom, present for approximately 2 months before MSCC occurs. The pain can be localised or progress to include radicular pain, usually becoming more severe over time (Al Qurainy & Collis, 2016). Metastases can affect any part of the spine but most commonly affects the thoracic (approximately 70%), followed by lumbar (20%), with the cervical being the least affected. Thirty percent are multi-level despite pain presenting at one site (Scuibba et al., 2010). Eighty five percent of MSCC is caused by haematogenous spread of the disease to the vertebral body which collapses and compresses the cord.

However, local tumour expansion into the spinal cord and metastatic deposits within the cord itself are also seen (Al Qurainy & Collis, 2016).

MSCC is a well-recognised complication of cancer and is usually an oncological emergency that requires early diagnosis and treatment to avoid permanent neurological consequences and paralysis. It is a complex and serious condition with devastating effects on the quality and the length of life remaining (Kwok et al., 2006). MSCC is defined as:

> *spinal cord or cauda equina compression by direct pressure and/or induction of vertebral collapse or instability by metastatic spread or direct extension of malignancy that threatens or causes neurological disability*

NICE, 2008

MSCC can occur in four distinct anatomical areas within the spinal cord:
- intramedullary, rare (within the spinal cord)
- extramedullary (outside the spinal cord)
- intradural (inside the dura)
- extradural (outside the dura)

In the latter stages of the disease, the tumour spread can invade the extradural space. The onset can be gradual or sudden (Kaplow & Iyere, 2016).

MSCC occurs when there is pathological vertebral body collapse or direct tumour growth causing compression of the spinal cord leading to irreversible neurological damage (Levack et al., 2002). Even thecal indentation (indentation of the sheath enclosing the spinal cord) by an extradural tumour mass is considered as MSCC (Loblaw & Laperrier, 1998). Bilsky et al. (2010) considered the reliability of analysis of spinal cord compression. In their study, they considered the reliability and validity of a magnetic resonance (MR) image-based grading system for epidural spinal cord compression (ESCC; Fig. 7.1) and produced a valid and reliable scale that may be used to describe the degree of ESCC based on T2-weighted MR images.

ESCC grading scale (Bilsky et al., 2010):

- 0 = bone disease only
- 1a = epidural impingement, without deformation of the thecal sac
- 1b = deformation of the thecal sac without spinal cord abutment
- 1c = deformation of the thecal sac with spinal cord abutment but without cord compression
- 2 = spinal cord compression but with cerebrospinal fluid (CSF) visible around the cord
- 3 = spinal cord compression, no CSF visible around the cord

In addition to the agonising pain and spinal instability that the condition can cause, compression of the spinal cord can also lead to paraplegia or quadriplegia and double incontinence. Alarming data from a seminal audit identified that, at diagnosis, 82% of patients with MSCC are unable to walk or only able to do so with help (Patchell et al., 2005). The development of paraplegia and loss of control of bladder and bowel function has a devastating effect on the quality of life that remains and considerably reduces life expectancy (Levack et al., 2002; Patchell et al., 2005). Those with established paraparesis and loss of bladder control by the time of treatment are unlikely to regain useful function (Christie, 2008).

Within the context of the very large numbers of people suffering from back pain (see Chapter 1 Introduction) and the relatively small numbers of these who have serious pathology, the challenges for diagnosis of serious

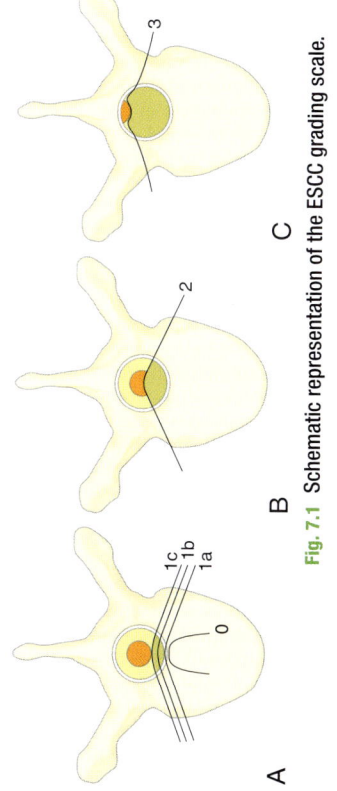

Fig. 7.1 Schematic representation of the ESCC grading scale.

TABLE 7.2 Three case studies highlighting differing levels of index of suspicion.

55-year-old female	55-year-old female	55-year-old female
Progressing back and leg pain to ankle Not responding to simple analgesics No history of cancer	Progressing back and leg pain to ankle Not responding to simple analgesics History of breast cancer 8 years ago	Progressing back and leg pain to ankle Not responding to simple analgesics Currently being treated for breast cancer

pathology cannot be underestimated. Early diagnosis depends on multiple factors. We rely on the patient presenting for medical advice early in the cancer disease process. Many patients report symptoms to a medical practitioner within 3 weeks of the onset of symptoms (Levack et al., 2001). It is significant that approximately 25% of cases presenting with MSCC will present with MSCC as the first sign of malignancy (NICE, 2008). This has great implications in clinical practice, particularly early in the disease pathway when symptoms are subtle and vague. Consider your 'index of suspicion' in the three case studies when investigating Red Flags during the subjective history (Table 7.2).

The history of breast cancer should significantly influence your clinical reasoning. So now stop for a moment and consider that approximately 25% of patients with MSCC do not even know that they have cancer, and so will not be reporting this to you. How does this influence your clinical reasoning? This scenario is commonly known as 'malignancy of undefined primary origin' (MUO) (NICE, 2010). The primary cancer is often identified subsequently following investigation; however, in some cases, despite extensive investigation, no primary can be confirmed. These patients are described as suffering from 'cancer of unknown primary' (CUP) (NICE, 2010). It must also be remembered that, on some occasions, there is a history of a known cancer but the metastases identified are from another unknown cancer, further adding to the clinical complexity of these cases. Frymoyer (1997) states *do not ignore any history of cancer;* however, it must be considered that a metastatic lesion may be from another primary altogether. An example of this is Bob, a 61-year-old man with a history of bladder cancer. He presented to an orthopaedic interface service with a new onset of back and leg pain, weakness in his legs and a wide-based gait. In addition, he suffered from significant sleep disturbance. MSCC was suspected and later confirmed; however, the primary cancer was in the lung.

Patients can present anywhere in the healthcare system but commonly present to a front-line generalist clinician in a primary or secondary care setting. If cancer metastasises to the spine, the gravity of the clinical picture can potentially escalate rapidly to a serious stage. Therefore, the earlier we can identify spinal malignancy, the better the length and quality of life remaining.

As discussed in the introductory chapter, early in the spinal malignancy disease process (prodromal phase) symptoms are often subtle and vague and so the ongoing collaboration between the patient and the clinician is of paramount importance in recognising if symptoms are developing a more sinister trend. Observing behaviour of symptoms over time using a 'watchful-wait' approach can be extremely helpful in identifying serious disease early in some cases (Cook et al., 2018). Over a period of time, a combination of Red Flags can become more apparent when a patient is closely monitored (Franci et al., 2016). Analysis of serious cases has also identified that, during a period of watchful waiting, consistency of clinician can be of further benefit to enhance the often overlooked clinical tool, clinical suspicion (Mitchell et al., 2012). To aid early diagnosis further, we rely on the clinician's communication skills and awareness of Red Flags. It is essential that clinicians possess the clinical skill to cue the patient into understanding early serious symptoms of spinal malignancy and actions to take should they develop. More studies are necessary to investigate communication involving all serious conditions including malignancy. Christina, recently diagnosed with multiple spinal and visceral metastases with an underlying history of breast cancer, illustrated her lack of understanding with the following extract taken from a one to one interview shortly after her diagnosis:

> *...I am very lucky it is treatable but not curable...at least it is not terminal!*

Early identification of spinal metastasis

If a patient is diagnosed with spinal malignancy at the point when there is one solitary tumour, the outcome is much more favourable. MSCC is often caused by vertebral collapse; hence, identification of a metastatic lesion early is key. However, as previously described, early symptoms can be subtle and vague with many patients presenting with painless spinal malignant lesions which are only identified when other sites prompt investigation.

Robson (2014) describes a list of Red Flags for MSCC; however, these tend to be features suggestive of late disease:

- limb weakness
- difficulty walking
- sensory loss
- bladder or bowel dysfunction
- neurological signs
- cervical or thoracic pain
- pain increased on straining
- night pain

According to Al Qurainy & Collis (2016), pain deteriorating over time, worse on coughing, sneezing, straining (Valsalva manoeuvre) or lying supine can suggest epidural distension.

More recently (2018, unpublished data), 21 advanced practitioners and medical consultants attending a National Back Pain Conference screening workshop were asked to consider the five most important items in screening for spinal malignancy. The participants were self-selecting having chosen the screening workshop. A qualitative methodology was employed using a short version nominal group technique (NGT) (McMillan et al., 2016). The NGT approach was chosen to generate themes for further consideration relating to screening for serious spinal conditions. The first stage required the delegates to complete blank post cards with their top five items for screening for spinal malignancy. During this first stage, delegates were not allowed to communicate with one another and worked in silence. The second stage involved all delegates volunteering one of their top five items in turn until all had delivered all documented items. Facilitators recorded each item on a flip chart. Items (which were often repeated by delegates) were recorded by the facilitator to illustrate a weighting or level of agreement. After the NGT, the facilitators of the workshops collaboratively conducted an informal table-top analysis of the findings. The focus of items was on well-known Red Flags. However, the top five Red Flags were all associated with advanced or late-stage disease suggestive of cord compression:

- unwell
- weight loss
- abnormal neurology
- bladder dysfunction
- bowel dysfunction

These findings highlight the need for improved widespread dissemination of early Red Flags suggestive of serious disease to enable impending cord compression to be identified more readily rather than at the late compressive stage (these are discussed more fully later):

- atypical pain (e.g. chest wall or rib pain)
- band-like pain
- escalating pain
- funny feelings in legs
- difficulty lying flat

The patient experience

In order that we can diagnose metastatic disease early not only do we need early Red Flags, but we need our patients to present to the clinical setting at the right time early in the disease process. You heard from Christina earlier. She was a 56-year-old woman with a history of breast cancer and chronic low back pain. She initially presented with a flare up of long-standing intermittent back pain that she described as not new but a familiar pain experienced in the past. In fact, she reported a 44-year history of this pain. Within a short period of time, the pain escalated and became band-like and worse at night. Despite pain being in the lumbar spine only, whole-spinal MRI identified multiple spinal metastatic lesions throughout the thoracic and lumbosacral spine (Fig. 7.2). Christina's case illustrates the challenges that we face with early diagnosis of spinal metastasis.

Christina felt frustrated that she perceived that she had not been warned of what signs and symptoms to look out for in the future following her breast cancer diagnosis.

Hindsight is a wonderful thing you get scared cos it's constantly on your mind if I am honest in hindsight it changed in September. I should have sought help earlier, I knew there was something wrong. I have been too scared to do anything with it...I got told nothing. They are pamphlet happy. There must have been a dozen. Don't give me a pamphlet tell me what to look out for. Just tell me. They should be sitting people down. It takes five minutes. Look out for A, B and C. If this happens ring the breast unit...or the GP. Tell me what to look out for and what to do if they {symptoms} develop...There are lots of different secondaries...if you don't know what to look out for...you can easily miss something...and it's not to scare them but make them aware. Sit people down! Don't give them a leaflet to take away.

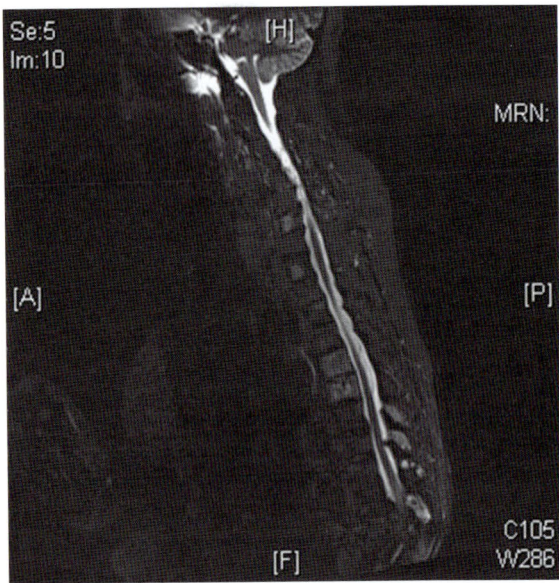

Fig. 7.2 Portion of Christina's whole spine MRI. The report describes metastatic deposits at T5, T6, T7, T10 and T11 vertebral bodies. The T11 vertebral body also shows metastatic deposits in the posterior elements bilaterally, predominantly on left side. The spinous process of T10 shows metastatic deposits. The T12 vertebral body and its posterior elements, predominantly on left side, are diffusely infiltrated by metastatic deposits. The L1 vertebral body is infiltrated by metastatic deposits predominantly along its right half and also involves the pedicles bilaterally. Metastatic infiltrative deposits are also seen at L2, L3, L4 and L5, and at sacral vertebrae.

Hutchison et al. (2012) identified that only 4% of staff interviewed reported giving any information about MSCC to patients at risk. In comparison, the same study highlighted that 77% of patients reported that they wanted information.

The following quotes have been taken from *When Breath Becomes Air* by Paul Kalinithi (2016). This is a true story of a 36-year-old neurosurgeon with spinal metastases and undiagnosed lung cancer. Even with his expert skills as a neurosurgeon, Paul struggled to identify the seriousness of his own symptoms as the condition waxed and waned:

The x-ray (flexion extension spinal x-ray) looked fine. We chalked the symptoms up to hard work and an aging body, scheduled a follow-up appointment and I went back to finishing my last case of the day. The weight loss slowed and the back pain became tolerable. A healthy dose of Ibuprofen got me through the day...

I could see the tension in my back unwind as my work schedule eased and life became more manageable

Over the past few months I'd had back spasms of varying ferocity, from simple ignorable pain, to pain that made me forsake speech to grind my teeth, to pain so severe I curled up on the floor screaming

I knew a lot about back pain—its anatomy, its physiology, the different words patients used to describe different kinds of pain—but I did not know what it felt like. Maybe that's all this was. Maybe.

As Paul observed his own symptoms over time, the situation changed:

> *Then a few weeks later I began having bouts of chest pain. Had I bumped into something at work? Cracked a rib somehow? Some nights I'd wake up on soaked sheets. Dripping sweat. My weight began dropping again, more rapidly now, from 175 to 145 pounds (79 to 66 Kg). I developed a persistent cough. Little doubt remained.*

Paul illustrates the classic fluctuation in symptoms early in the disease process which often contributes to the diagnosis being delayed.

Risk factors for MSCC

The literature to date lacks evidence relating to combinations of Red Flags for specific conditions and metastatic risk for those who have suffered from cancer. Sutcliffe et al. (2013) undertook a systematic review to examine the natural history of spinal metastases with progress to MSCC. They estimated the mean survival as between 3 and 7 months with the probability of survival at 12 months as 36%. Their review suggested that risk of vertebral fracture and resultant spinal cord compression depended on a number of factors. The higher the number of spinal metastases and the longer they were present for, then the higher the risk of spinal cord compression; risk was further increased if spread included bony lesions. Prostate cancer studies identified that tumour grade, metastatic load and duration on hormone therapy increased risk of MSCC. There was a greater risk with a Gleason score greater than or equal to 7 (Table 7.3). Six or more bone lesions produced a higher risk than those with less than

TABLE 7.3 Risk factors for MSCC in prostate cancer.

Prostate cancer (risk of future metastatic disease at diagnosis)	
High Gleason score more than or equal to 8 regardless of prostate-specific antigen (PSA)	Gleason score is a system of grading prostate cancer based on the investigation of affected tissue under a microscope. Gleason scores range from 2 to 10 and indicate how likely spread of the disease is A low score (grade 1) suggests that the prostate tissue looks similar to normal prostate cells; therefore, it is less likely to spread. Grade 5 is the highest score. If the score is high, the tissue is very different from that of a normal prostate with a higher propensity to spread. Prostate cancers often have areas of different grades. A grade is assigned to the two areas that make up the bulk of the cancer growth. These two grades are added together to produce the Gleason score. The first number is the grade for the largest area e.g. 4 + 3 = 7 (American Cancer Society, 2017)
High PSA at diagnosis more than or equal to 50	PSA is a protein excreted by the prostate gland. A PSA of 4.0 ng/mL and below has been considered as normal. However, this must not be used in isolation as some with low PSA have been found to have prostate cancer and vice versa. However, in general, the higher the PSA score, the more concerning the results. Experts felt that a PSA equal to or above 50 at diagnosis is a risk factor of future metastatic activity (National Cancer Institute, 2017)

TABLE 7.3 Risk factors for MSCC in prostate cancer.—cont'd

Patient with relapsed disease	This appears straightforward but the patient may not know that the disease has recurred. In a patient with a history of prostate cancer and newly developed back pain, close monitoring over time is essential to enable intervention with timely and appropriate investigations. An important scenario to consider is that the patient may have a history of cancer but the original cancer is not actually producing metastasis in the spine! You will remember Bob (mentioned earlier), with a previous history of bladder cancer. Although bladder cancer is not well known to metastasise to the spine, Bob's presenting symptoms were concerning and the MSCC pathway was instigated and an emergency whole-spine MRI organised that day. Bob did have MSCC but the primary cancer was an undiagnosed primary lesion in the lung

six bone lesions. The same systematic review for breast cancer patients identified four variables important in identifying MSCC risk (Table 7.4): bone metastasis less than 2 years, metastatic disease at initial diagnosis, objective neurological deficit and vertebral compression fracture.

In an endeavour to improve identification of spinal metastases early in a generalist primary care setting, a group of experts in the field of oncology and palliative care in the north west of England were asked their opinion about the risk of developing spinal metastatic disease relating to the three cancers that most commonly

TABLE 7.4 Risk factors for MSCC in breast cancer.

Breast cancer (risk of future metastatic disease at diagnosis)	
High-grade disease (grade 3)	Some types of cancer have their own grading systems but generally there are 3 grades: Grade 1—The cancer cells look very similar to normal cells and are growing slowly Grade 2—The cancer cells look unlike normal cells and are growing more quickly than normal Grade 3—The cancer cells look very abnormal and are growing quickly Some systems have more than 3 grades GX means that the grade cannot be assessed. It is also called undetermined grade (Cancer Research UK, 2017a)
Tumour T3 or above	TNM staging takes into account the size of the tumour (T), whether the cancer has spread to the lymph nodes (N), and whether the tumour has spread anywhere else in the body (M—for metastases) T1—the tumour is 2 cm in diameter or less T2—the tumour is more than 2 cm but less than 5 cm T3—the tumour is bigger than 5 cm in diameter (Cancer Research UK, 2017b)
Triple negative cancers (ER, PgR, HER-2 neg)	Triple negative breast cancer is a type of breast cancer that does not have receptors for oestrogen and progesterone or the protein HER-2. These are more common in women under 40 and black women. Some women with this type of cancer have the faulty BRACA1 gene (MacMillan, 2016a)

TABLE 7.4 Risk factors for MSCC in breast cancer.—cont'd

HER-2 breast positive cancer	HER-2 is known as human epidermal growth factor and is a protein that can affect the growth of certain cancer cells and is found on the surface of normal breast tissue. In some cases, the breast cancer cell has a large proportion of HER-2 receptors. These extra receptors can stimulate the division and growth of cancer cells. Between 15% and 25% of breast cancers fall into this category. These cancers tend to grow more rapidly than HER-negative breast cancer (MacMillan, 2016b)
Node-positive cancer	Node-positive breast cancer means that cancer cells from the tumour in the breast have been identified in the lymph nodes

metastasise to bone including the spine. This as yet unpublished data could prove very informative for the generalist clinician. The following question was used as a prompt for this exercise:

> *Should the patients know that they have had, or have cancer, what information could help to inform our {generalist clinician} index of suspicion?*

This group of oncology and palliative care clinicians highlighted that it is worth remembering that 'low-risk' ER (oestrogen receptor)+ cancers can relapse with bony metastases (thus high risk of MSCC) 5–10 years after initial diagnosis but 'high-risk' cancers usually relapse within 3–5 years of initial diagnosis. The oncology experts felt that there was no obvious 'high-risk' group for developing metastases at diagnosis of lung cancer. Diagnosis of lung cancer alone was the biggest risk factor. See Table 7.3 for a list of risk factors for MSCC in prostate cancer and Table 7.4 for a list of risk factors for MSCC in breast cancer.

Although breast, prostate and lung cancers are known to commonly metastasise to the spine, it must be borne in mind that in a situation with patients living longer, any solid tumour cancer, for example colorectal, can lead to MSCC, along with haematological cancers such as myeloma and lymphoma.

Diagnosis of MSCC

The issue of identifying MSCC early by recognising subtle signs, to prevent serious long-term disability, was a key theme identified by the task and finish group at Greater Manchester and Cheshire Cancer Network (GMCCN) in 2009. It was this group who coordinated the development of credit card-sized cue cards for clinicians as part of their strategic approach to improving care for MSCC patients (Turnpenny et al., 2013). A variety of stakeholder groups identified a credit card format as a quick, visually attractive way of helping to promote key clinical messages and to raise awareness of particular health issues across a broad range of professionals. The GMCCN used their strategic position to bring together the oncology expertise and primary care musculoskeletal physiotherapy expertise to work on producing a user-friendly list of MSCC Red Flags for non-specialist 'generalist' front-line clinicians working in primary care settings.

Three key statements about MSCC were formulated, along with signposting to key sources of additional information (https://www.nice.org.uk):

- past medical history of cancer (but note 25% of patients do not have diagnosed primary)
- early diagnosis is essential (as the prognosis is severely impaired once paralysis occurs)
- a combination of Red Flags increases suspicion (the more Red Flags, the higher the risk and the greater urgency)

In addition, a user-friendly list of Red Flags for MSCC was agreed, which was then developed into an 8-item Red Flag mnemonic (Fig. 7.3) (Turnpenny et al., 2013).

The objective examination will only reveal abnormalities with more advanced disease but essentially needs to be thorough not only for the diagnostic process, but to give a baseline for disease progression. A structured chronological sequence of examination is suggested to thoroughly examine the integrity of each spinal level including the integrity of the spinal nerves and the spinal cord.

The following figure (Fig. 7.4) is taken from West of Scotland Guidelines for Malignant Spinal Cord Compression (West of Scotland Cancer Network, 2013).

Although many MSCC guidelines do not mention reflex testing, within musculoskeletal practice, reflex testing can give additional information, for example brisk, absent or, in the case of the plantar and Hoffman responses, positive findings. The plantar response, sometimes known as the Babinski response, is an important neurologic examination. The lateral aspect of the foot is stroked and the action of the big toe is observed. An upward-going big toe gives cause for concern relating to an upper motor neurone lesion. The Hoffmann sign is elicited by flicking the nail of the third finger. Flexion of the ipsilateral thumb and/or

▌ BOX 7.1 Frankel classification.

A – Absence of motor or sensory function below the level of the lesion

B – Absence of motor function, but with some degree of sensitivity preserved below the level of the lesion

C – Some degree of motor function but without practical usefulness

D – Useful motor function below the level of the lesion

E – Normal sensory and motor function, although there may be some abnormality of reflexes

finger is a positive sign. Careful documentation of the findings of each test is essential to facilitate speed of progress of the disease and monitor signs of cord compression.

Once MSCC is suspected, the gold standard investigation is a whole spinal MRI. If the image is suggestive of MSCC, and particularly if there is no known primary cancer, further investigations are required, such as staging computerised tomography (CT) to establish the ultimate diagnosis. This is often carried out by the specialist oncology team.

There are a number of classification systems in use once MSCC has been identified. One of these is the 5-level Frankel classification system based on initial neurological status (Franic et al., 2016) (Box 7.1).

Difficulty in differentiating between pain from spinal metastasis and pain from MSCC is well recognised. NICE (2008) recommends whole-spine MRI as the gold standard investigation to help to differentiate between these two very different states. For those with spinal metastasis pain alone, MRI within 7 days is accepted. For those with pain and neurological deficit (MSCC), 24 hours is the investigation window of choice. MRI has a sensitivity of 93% and a specificity

Red Flags

EARLY WARNING SIGNS OF MSCC
Greenhalgh S, Turnpenney J, Richards L, Selfe J (2010)

R   Referred back pain is <u>multi</u>-segmental or <u>band-like</u>

E   <u>Escalating pain</u> which is poorly responsive to treatment (incl medication)

D   <u>Different</u> character or site to previous symptoms

F   <u>Funny</u> feelings, odd sensations or <u>heavy legs</u> (multi-segmental)

L   <u>Lying</u> flat increases back pain

A   <u>Agonising</u> pain causing anguish and despair

G   <u>Gait</u> disturbance, unsteadiness, especially on stairs (not just a limp)

S   <u>Sleep</u> grossly disturbed due to pain being worse at night

NB – Established motor/sensory/bladder/bowel disturbances → late signs

Red Flags

Referred or BAND-LIKE pain
Escalating Pain: Poor response to treatment
Different character or site than previous

Funny or 'odd sensations' or 'heavy legs'
Lying flat increases pain
Agonising or severe back pain
Gait disturbance: Unsteady, stairs difficult
Sleep disturbance with night pain

Established Motor/Sensory/Bladder/Bowel disturbances are LATE SIGNS = poor functional outcome and survival.

Fig. 7.3 MSCC credit card with Red Flag mnemonic.

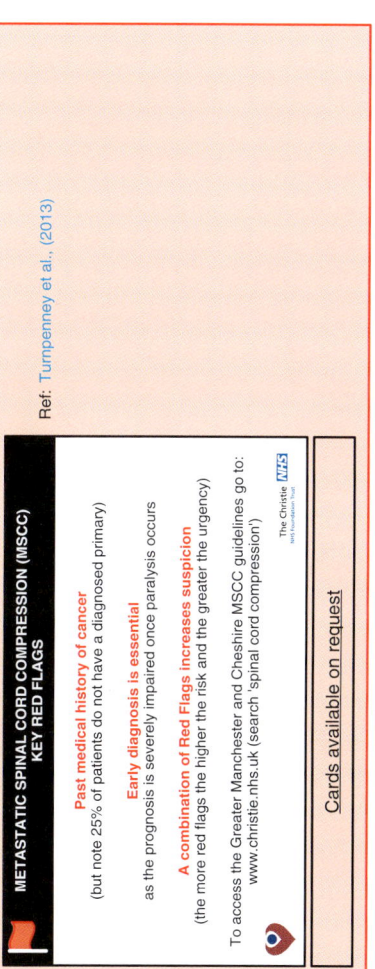

METASTATIC SPINAL CORD COMPRESSION (MSCC)
KEY RED FLAGS

Past medical history of cancer
(but note 25% of patients do not have a diagnosed primary)

Early diagnosis is essential
as the prognosis is severely impaired once paralysis occurs

A combination of Red Flags increases suspicion
(the more red flags the higher the risk and the greater the urgency)

To access the Greater Manchester and Cheshire MSCC guidelines go to:
www.christie.nhs.uk (search 'spinal cord compression')

The Christie NHS
NHS Foundation Trust

Cards available on request

Ref: Turnpenney et al., (2013)

Fig. 7.3, cont'd

Sensation–key levels

C4   Shoulders
C6   Thumbs
T10   Umbilicus
T12   Groin
L3   Front of knee
L5   Big toe
S1   Little toe
S3   Genitalia

Muscle power–
Muscle groups are charted using the Oxford classification

0 = Complete paralysis
1 = Flicker of contraction
2 = Contraction with gravity eliminated
3 = Contraction against gravity
4 = Contraction against gravity and resistance (weaker than normal)
5 = Normal contraction

Fig. 7.4 Components of objective examination for MSCC.

Muscle groups nerve roots

Upper limb

C3 (4)	Trapezius
C5	Deltoid
C5 (6)	Biceps
C6 (7, 8)	Pectorals
C6 (7, 8)	Wrist extensors
C7 (8)	Finger extensors
C7 (8)	Wrist flexors
C7 (8)	Triceps
C8 (T1)	Finger flexors
T1	Interossei

Lower limb

L1 (2)	Hip flexors
L3 (4)	Quadriceps
L4 (5), S1	Dorsi-flexors & hip
	Abductors
L2 (3)	Hip Adductors
L5,S1	Internal & external
	rotators
	Hamstrings
S1 (2)	Plantar flexors
L5, S1, S2	Gluteals

Trunk

T6-L1	Abdominals
C1-L5	Back extensors

Fig. 7.4, cont'd

Muscle tone—

To quantify increased tone, the modified Ashworth Scale can be used

4 = Rigidity

3 = Movement difficult, considerable tone

2 = More marked increase in tone, still easily moved

1+ = Slight increase in tone, catch and resistance throughout range of movement

1 = Slight increase in tone, catch and minimum resistance at end of range

0 = No increase in tone

Fig. 7.4, cont'd

of 97%. A small number (7%) will have a diagnosis missed on MRI and an even smaller number (3%) will have a false positive. CT is used to assist surgical or radiotherapy preparation and not recommended for definitive diagnosis unless MRI is contraindicated (Al-Qurainy & Collis, 2016). One of the other recommendations from NICE in its key priorities for effective management of MSCC was the appointment of an MSCC coordinator who would act as a single point of access for clinicians (NICE, 2008). This role encompasses the coordination of timely onward management of MSCC patients, which includes advice and management, along a clear pathway based on up-to-date evidence. The next chapter describes one such MSCC pathway; however, it is vitally important that readers of this book are prepared for the '4.00 pm on a Friday' scenario and acquaint themselves with their own local MSCC pathway whether they are practising in Honolulu or Hull.

References

Al-Qurainy R, Collis E. Metastatic spinal cord compression; diagnosis and management. *BMJ*. 2016;353(i2539):1–7.

American Cancer Society. *Understanding Your Pathology Report: Prostate Cancer*; 2017. http://www.cancer.org/treatment/understanding-your-diagnosis/tests/understanding-your-pathology-report/prostate-pathology/prostate-cancer-pathology.html.

Bilsky M, Laufer I, Fourney D, et al. Reliability analysis of the epidural spinal cord compression scale. *J Neurosurg Spine*. 2010;13:324–328.

Brooks F, Ghatahora A, Brooks M, et al. Management of metastatic spinal cord compression; awareness of NICE guidance. *Eur J Orthop Surg Traumatol*. 2014;24(Suppl 1):S255–S259.

Cancer Research UK. *Cancer Grading*. 2017a. http://www.cancerresearchuk.org/about-cancer/what-is-cancer/cancer-grading#common.

Cancer Research UK. *TNM Staging for Breast Cancer*. 2017b. http://www.cancerresearchuk.org/about-cancer/type/breast-cancer/treatment/tnm-breast-cancer-staging#what.

Christie Hospital NHS Foundation Trust. *Spinal Cord Compression Guidelines*. Manchester; 2008.

Coleman R, Holen I. *Chapter 51, Bone Metastases*. 5th ed. Elsevier inc; 2014.

Cook C, George S, Reiman, M. Red Flag screening for low back pain: nothing to see here, move along: a narrative review. *Br J Sports Med*. 2017; 52(8);52:493–496.

Ellis-Brookes L, McPhail S, Ives A, et al. Routes to diagnosis for cancer; determining the patient journey using multiple routine dataset. *Br J Cancer*. 2012;107(8):1220–1226.

Franic M, Bilic V, Dokuzovic S, Curic S, Cengic T, Rotim K. Surgical treatment of metastatic disease of the vertebral column. *Acta Clin Croat*. 2016;55(3):474–482.

Frymoyer JW. *The Adult Spine: Principles and Practice*. Lippincott-Raven Publishers; 1997.

Hartvigsen J, Hancock M, Kongsted A, et al. Low Back Pain 1: what low back pain is and why we need to pay attention. Lancet low Back Pain Series Working Group. *Lancet*. 2018;391:P2356–2367.

Hutchison C, Morrison A, Rice AM, Tait G, Harden S. Provision of information about malignant spinal cord compression; perceptions of patients and staff. *Int J Palliat Nurs*. 2012;(2):61–68.

Kalinithi P. *When Breath Becomes Air*. Vintage Publishing; 2016.

Kaplow R, Iyere K. Oncology emergency series. Understanding spinal cord compression. *Nursing*. 2016;46(9):44–50.

Kwok Y, Tibbs PA, Patchell RA. Clinical approach to meta-static epidural spinal cord compression. *Hematol Oncol Clin North Am*. 2006;20:1297–1305.

Levack P, Graham J, Collie D, et al. *A Prospective Audit of the Diagnosis, Management and Outcome of Malignant Cord Compression (CRAG 97/08)*. Edinburgh: CRAG. West of Scotland NHS; 2001.

Levack P, Graham J, Collie D, et al. Don't wait for a sensory level-listen to the symptoms: a prospective audit of the delays in diagnosis of malignant cord compression. *Clin Oncol*. 2002;14:472–480.

Loblaw D, Laperrier N. Emergency treatment of malignant extradural spinal cord compression: an evidence-based guideline. *J Clin Oncol*. 1998;16(4):1613–1624.

Macmillan. Triple negative breast cancer. http://www.macmillan.org. uk/information-and-support/breast-cancer/understanding-cancer/types-of-breast-cancer/triple-negative-breast-cancer.html. 2016a.

Macmillan. HER-2 breast positive cancer. https://www.macmillan.org. uk/information-and-support/breast-cancer/understanding-cancer/types-of-breast-cancer/her-2-positive-breast-cancer.html. 2016b.

McMillan S, King M, Tully M. *How to Use Nominal Group Technique and Delphi Techniques. Int J Clin Pharm.* 2016;38(3):655–662.

Mitchell E, Rubin G, Macleod U. *Improving Diagnosis; A Toolkit for General Practice.* 2012.

National Cancer Institute. *Prostate-Specific Antigen (PSA) Test.* 2017. https://www.cancer.gov/types/prostate/psa-fact-sheet#q3.

NICE. Metastatic Malignant disease of unknown primary origin in adults; diagnosis and management (CG104). 2010. www.nice.org.uk/guidance/cg104.

NICE. Metastatic spinal cord compression in adults: risk assessment, diagnosis and management Clinical guideline [CG75] (2008). 2008. https://www.nice.org.uk/Guidance/CG75.

Office for National Statistics. Geographic patterns of cancer survival in England: Adults diagnosed 2003 to 2010 and followed up to 2015. 2017. https://www.ons.gov.uk/peoplepopulationandcommunity/healthandsocialcare/conditionsanddiseases/bulletins/geographicpatternsofcancersurvivalinengland/adultsdiagnosed2003to2010andfollowedupto2015#geographic-patterns-of-cancer-survival.

Patchell R, Tibbs P, Regine W, et al. Direct decompressive surgical resection in the treatment of spinal cord compression caused by metastatic cancer: a randomised trial. *Lancet.* 2005;366:643–648.

Ponti A, et al. *Cancer Screening in the European Union: Report on the implementation of the Council Recommendation on Cancer Screening.* 2017. https://ec.europa.eu/health/sites/health/files/major_chronic_diseases/docs/2017_cancerscreening_2ndreportimplementation_en.pdf.

Robson P. Metastatic spinal cord compression: a rare but important complication of cancer. *Clin Med (Lond).* 2014;(5):542–545.

Sciubba D, Petteys R, Dekutoski M, et al. Diagnosis and management of metastatic spine disease a review. *J Neurosurg: Spine.* 2010;13(1):94–108.

Sutcliffe P, Connock M, Shyangdan D, Court R, Kandala NB, Clarke A. A systematic review of evidence on malignant spinal metastases: natural history and technologies for identifying patients at high risk of vertebral fracture and spinal cord compression. *Health Technol Assess.* 2013;17(42):1–274.

Turnpenney J, Greenhalgh S, Richards L, Crabtree A, Selfe J. Developing an early alert system for metastatic spinal cord compression. *Prim Health Care Res Dev.* 2013;16(1):14–20.

Tsukada Y, Nakamura N, Ohde S, Akahane K, Sekiguchi K, Terahara A. Factors that delay treatment of symptomatic metastatic extradural spinal cord compression. *J Palliat Med.* 2015;(2):107–113.

West of Scotland Cancer Network. *West of Scotland Guidelines for Malignant Spinal Cord Compression (V2).* 2013.

CHAPTER **8**

Metastatic Spinal Cord Compression (MSCC): Consequences and Care

As discussed in Chapter 7, in 25% of cases, metastatic spinal cord compression (MSCC) is the first manifestation of malignancy; metastases are well known to be an indicator of significant tumour progression associated with mortality and substantial morbidity. This late presentation limits the time for diagnostic workup. As a consequence, urgent treatment is often required before the primary tumour diagnosis (Wanman et al., 2017). Metastatic disease can result in end-organ failure through compression of various vital organs along with the spinal cord. MSCC is therefore a potentially life-changing oncological emergency. In such cases, immediate medical attention is required to maintain and restore neurological function, relieve pain and avoid permanent damage. Neurological function and quality of life can be preserved if patients receive an early diagnosis and rapid access to treatment to prevent or reduce nerve damage and to maintain spinal stability (Bowers, 2015). Substantial progress has been made in the management of MSCC in the last two decades. In 2001, the Clinical Resource and Audit Group (CRAG) report (Levack et al., 2001) identified significant delays from initial presentation to a medical practitioner to ultimate diagnosis.

This seminal report highlighted that approximately 82% of patients were unable to walk at this point (Levack et al., 2001), and marked a turning point in the approach to MSCC. According to White (2016), prognosis and outcome in MSCC depend on two main factors:

- ambulatory status at diagnosis
- primary tumour

National Institute for Health and Care Excellence (NICE, 2008), in their quick reference guide, summarise key priorities in the management of MSCC as follows (Table 8.1).

More recently, Robson (2014) confirms a series of practical steps to take:

- safety net those at risk of MSCC (i.e. those at high risk of bone metastases or those with bone metastases)
- whole spine magnetic resonance imaging (MRI) within 1 week for those spinal pain patients who have a diagnosis of cancer whose symptoms are suggestive of metastasis
- urgent whole spine MRI within 24 hours for those presenting with suggestion of MSCC and follow local MSCC pathway
- once MSCC confirmed, contact MSCC coordinator
- definitive treatment begins within 24 hours of MSCC confirmation

Despite these guidelines, an audit of 96 trainee doctors by Brooks et al. (2014) identified that MSCC was poorly understood and suggested that a greater understanding of the NICE guidelines is required to enhance MSCC management.

MSCC service configuration

Robust MSCC pathways with rapid access to assessment, investigation, diagnosis and treatment to improve patient

TABLE 8.1 NICE quick reference guide key priorities in the management of MSCC.

Service config-uration and urgency of treatment	Every cancer network should ensure appropriate patient-centred services are available to facilitate early diagnosis, treatment, rehabilitation and ongoing care for MSCC sufferers
Early detection	Contact MSCC coordinator immediately to discuss patients causing clinical concern relating to MSCC who present with the following:
	1. Neurological symptoms including radicular pain, limb weakness, gait disturbance, sensory loss or bladder or bowel dysfunction
	2. Neurological signs of cord or cauda equina compression (see cauda equina Chapter 5)
	Imaging
	Contact MSCC coordinator within 24 hours to discuss patients causing clinical concern relating to MSCC who present with a combination of the following:
	1. Thoracic or cervical pain
	2. Progressive lumbar pain
	3. Severe unremitting lumbar pain
	4. Pain aggravated by straining (Valsalva manoeuvre, cough, sneeze)
	5. Localised tenderness
	6. Night pain preventing sleep
	Whole spine MRI if MSCC suspected unless contraindicated within 24 hours (sooner if clinical need for emergency surgery)
	Safety net those patients at high risk of developing bone metastasis, i.e. patients known to have bone metastases or patients with cancer who present with spinal pain, educate them about MSCC symptoms
	MRI within 7 days if spinal malignancy suspected

TABLE 8.1 NICE quick reference guide key priorities in the management of MSCC.—cont'd	
Treatment of spinal metastases and MSCC	Suspected MSCC patients should be nursed flat until bony and neurological stability are confirmed (bespoke local pathways should be developed)
	Start definitive treatment if appropriate ideally within 24 hours of MSCC confirmation
	Surgical decision
	Ensure access within 24 hours to radiotherapy 7 days a week for MSCC sufferers requiring definitive treatment or who are unsuitable for surgery
Supportive care and rehabilitation	Rehabilitation and discharge planning should begin on admission. Planning should include patient, family and carers, oncology and rehabilitation team, community support and primary care and specialist palliative care teams as appropriate

outcomes are essential (Savage et al., 2014). One of the recommendations from NICE (2008) was the appointment of an MSCC coordinator who would act as a single point of access for clinicians. Their role encompasses the coordination of timely onward management of MSCC patients, which includes advice and management, along a clear pathway based on up-to-date evidence. Savage et al. (2014) highlight the CRAG report (Levack et al., 2001), which reported that patients had often suffered back pain for 3 months prior to diagnosis. Delays in diagnosis and treatment were found partly through a lack of 24-hour emergency MRI facilities. Organisational changes, such as the development of a 'hotline' for MSCC referrals to facilitate and expedite management, were found to improve outcomes, including better ambulatory status which is of paramount importance. Savage et al. (2014) considered the impact of NICE guidelines (2008) in the south west of England. Overall, the outcomes of cancer patients with MSCC were significantly improved compared with outcomes in the 1990s. Nevertheless, large numbers of cancer patients with MSCC will already have developed major neurological changes even before entering the MSCC pathway. Approximately 20% had no previous diagnosis of cancer and many with a pre-existing cancer diagnosis do not seek medical attention for new symptoms until significant neurological deficit was established. Savage et al. (2014) suggest that a public awareness campaign may help overcome this challenge and they confirm that more robust patient pathways are still needed to optimise outcomes by enhancing easy access to diagnosis, appropriate timely investigations and treatment.

The results from one of the largest cancer treatment centres in Europe, the Christie National Health Service (NHS) Foundation Trust MSCC coordinator service in the north west of England, have been very encouraging and confirm that collaborative work across boundaries impacts positively on patient overall survival (Richards et al., 2016). However, as yet unpublished data from this service identifies that only 13%–20% of MSCC cases are suitable surgical candidates. This is in line with published data that confirm that, of the 10%–20% of identified patients with cancer, 10%–20% develop neural compression possibly requiring surgical intervention (Fox et al., 2017). Other studies conducted within the Christie MSCC coordinator service confirm that communication has been facilitated between the local primary and secondary care services with the tertiary specialist treating centre. Most patients presenting with MSCC received radiotherapy within 24 hours and the number of patients discussed with the surgical team increased threefold (Richards et al., 2016). The pivotal paper that identified surgery as giving the best outcome for functional performance and prognosis, Patchell et al. (2005), identified the median survival of MSCC patients post-surgery was 126 days. This compares to a post-radiotherapy median survival of approximately 30 days. Fehlings et al. (2016) reported the median survival of their MSCC patients in the USA and Canada as 234 days. Christie statistics identify a post-radiotherapy mean survival of 62 days compared with a post-surgery mean survival of 377 days. If surgery had not been available, these patients would have suffered more or would have had a premature death. The initial conclusion drawn was that a coordinated MSCC service has led to an increase in awareness in both health professionals and patients resulting in earlier diagnosis and treatment and improved survival. This type of pathway model, bespoke to the locality and suggested by NICE (2008), can be replicated across boundaries in many healthcare settings.

A local bespoke MSCC guide to management at the acute MSCC stage may look something like this (Fig. 8.1):

In this particular management strategy, as soon as suspicion of MSCC is raised, the MSCC coordinator is contacted and the patient nursed flat (Fig. 8.1). The patient would then be transported by ambulance, remaining flat, to the local District General Hospital. At that stage, further assessment and investigations would take place, including a whole spinal MRI and the administration of steroids. From a primary care perspective, this initial management is important to understand. There is likely to be a locally agreed pathway bespoke to the particular geographical area. Some multidisciplinary teams (MDT) may agree not to nurse flat so early in the pathway. Ensuring you have knowledge of what your locally agreed pathway

Immediate management of suspected MSCC

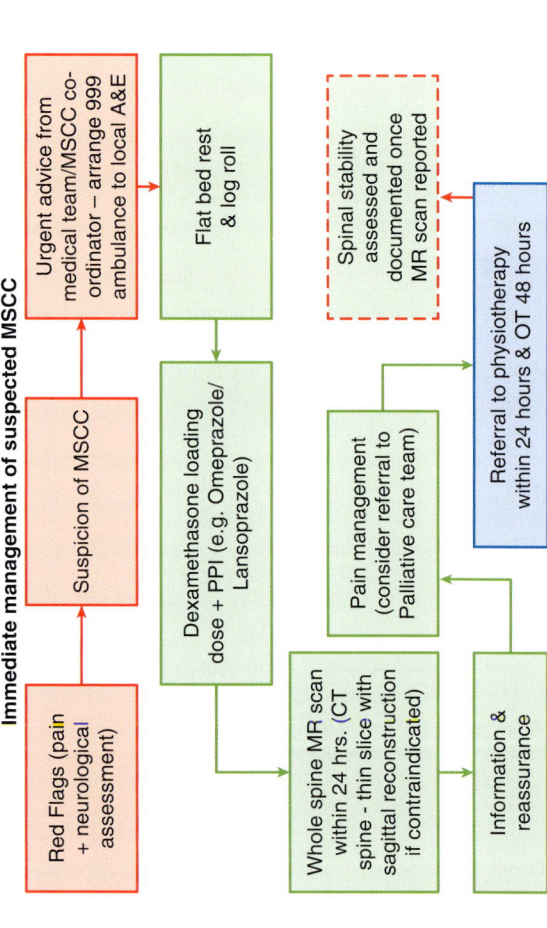

Fig. 8.1 **Immediate management of suspected MSCC.** *A&E,* Accident & Emergency; *CT,* computed tomography; *MRI,* magnetic resonance imaging; *MSCC,* metastatic spinal cord compression; *OT,* occupational therapy; *PPI,* proton pump inhibitor.

recommends or requires is essential. The current local pathway linked to this management strategy is highlighted below (Fig. 8.2).

Spinal stability

If the spinal column is affected by metastatic disease, there is a potential for spinal instability with consequent risk of neurological damage due to movement of the affected spinal segment (Table 8.2). Therefore, a strict nursing regime is of paramount importance in the management of MSCC (Kaplow & Iyere, 2016). The clinical decision relating to spinal stability remains a difficult decision and consequently is a multi-disciplinary judgement. To complicate the situation further, as the condition is a dynamic process with likely tumour growth, a stable spine can become unstable as a result of minor trauma or tumour expansion. Consequently, regular neurological status update and patient safety netting is important. The stability decision has a direct impact on mobilisation of the sufferer of MSCC and so is of vital importance to both patient and clinician. Pease et al. (2004) is the only study cited as examining timing of mobilisation and influence on patient outcome. Pease et al. (2004) identified that early mobilisation following confirmation of spinal stability reduces complication rates and has a direct impact on survival at 60 weeks. As mentioned earlier in Chapter 6, evidence suggests that only 10% of MSCC sufferers will progress to spinal instability but establishing who these 10% are is the critical factor.

Current practice also considers the spinal instability neoplastic score (SINS) (Fisher et al., 2010). The SINS was developed as a prognostic tool to aid the assessment of

TABLE 8.2 MSCC spinal stability indicators.

Site of disease	Cervical spine least stable, thoracic spine most stable due to added support of ribs and chest wall
Extent of tumour infiltration	Collapsed vertebrae are less likely to be stable especially if less than 50% of original height
Comorbidity	Pre-existing osteoporosis
Effect of open surgery	Spinal decompression may alter the stability of the spinal fixation
Disease progression	Tumour expansion
Radiological evidence	MRI and CT essential components in stability assessment to identify site, lytic lesion, structural deformity, alignment and posterolateral involvement
Clinical symptoms	Severe pain at site of lesion, pain increasing on movement, worsening neurology

patients with a spinal malignancy. It was developed by the Spinal Oncology Study Group (SOSG) in 2010 (Fisher et al., 2010). The SINS score is a reliable tool for spinal surgeons, radiologists and radiology oncologists which identifies those patients who are potentially suitable for surgical intervention (Fox et al., 2017). It assesses six variables, providing each with a score (Table 8.3):

Score 0–6: stable spine

Score 7–12: indeterminate, possible impending instability

Score 13–18: instability

Scores of more than 7 indicate that a spinal surgical opinion is recommended (Fox et al., 2017).

The spinal stability decision is ultimately taken by an MDT with input from the spinal team when appropriate.

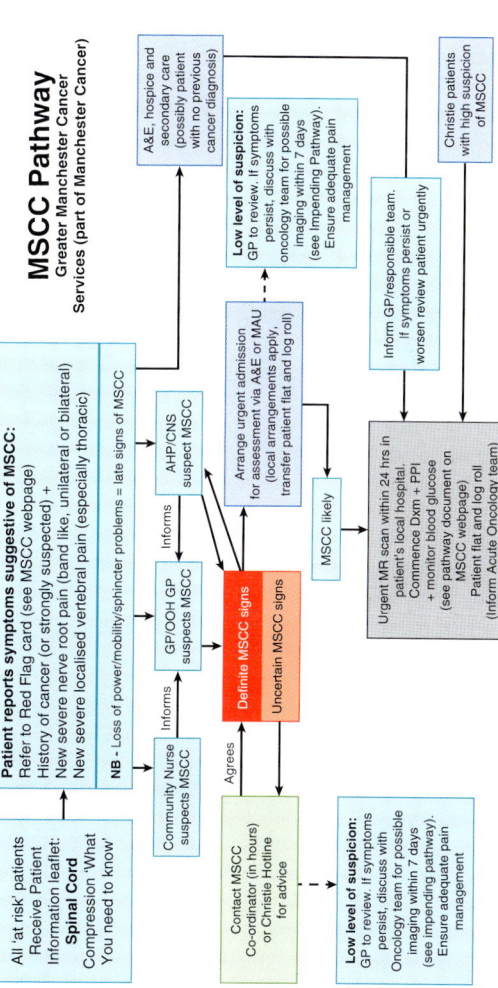

Fig. 8.2 Manchester Cancer MSCC Pathway. Available on the Christie NHS FT web site (http://www.christie.nhs.uk). *A&E*, Accident & Emergency; *AHP*, allied health professional; *CNS*, central nervous system; *DXM*, dextromethorphan, *FT*, Foundation Trust; *GP*, general practitioner; *MAU*, medical assessment unit; *MRI*, magnetic resonance imaging; *MSCC*, metastatic spinal cord compression; *OOH*, out-of-hours; *PPI*, proton pump inhibitor; *XRT*, radiotherapy.

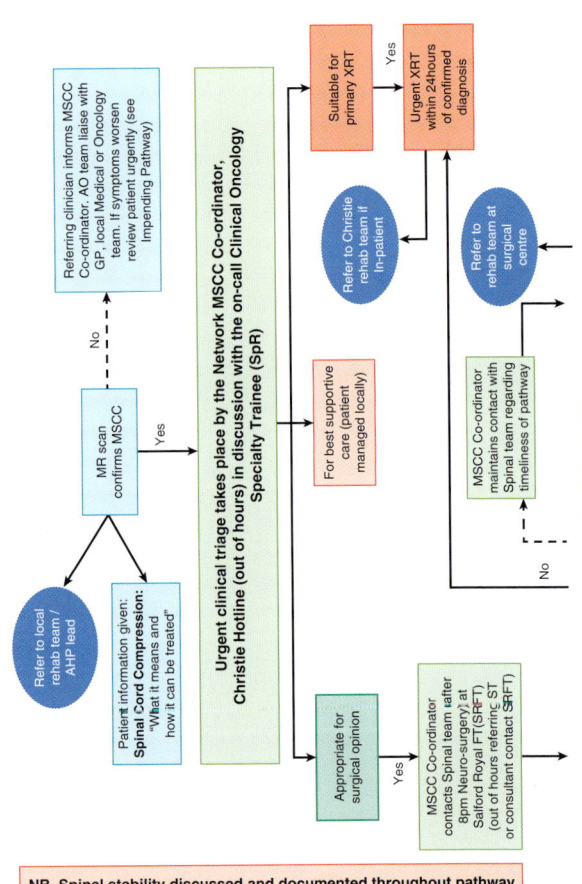

Fig. 8.2, cont'd

NB. Spinal stability discussed and documented throughout pathway

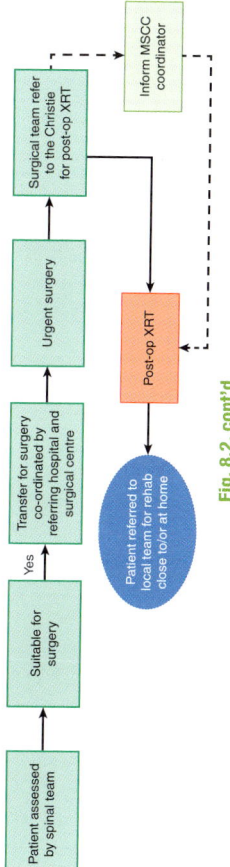

Fig. 8.2, cont'd

TABLE 8.3 SINS scores.

SINS Component	Score
Location	
Junctional (occiput–C2, C7–T2, T11–L1, L5–S1)	3
Mobile spine (C3–C6, L2–L4)	2
Semirigid (T3–T10)	1
Rigid (S2–S5)	0
Pain*	
Yes	3
Occasional pain but not mechanical	1
Pain-free lesion	0
Bone lesion	
Lytic	2
Mixed (lytic/blastic)	1
Blastic	0
Radiographic spinal alignment	
Subluxation/translation present	4
De novo deformity (kyphosis/scoliosis)	2
Normal alignment	0
Vertebral body collapse	
>50% collapse	3
<50% collapse	2
No collapse with >50% body involved	1
None of the above	0
Posterolateral involvement of spinal elements†	
Bilateral	3
Unilateral	1
None of the above	0

Note: Data adapted.
SINS, Spinal instability neoplastic score.
*Pain improvement with recumbency and/or pain with movement/loading of spine.
†Facet, pedicle or costovertebral joint fracture or replacement with tumour.

Timely input into the decision is required from a radiologist and medical team along with the physiotherapy team. A combination of factors offers the best clinical guide to this decision-making process:

- clinical features
- mechanical pain
- deterioration in neurology
- radiological findings

NICE (2008) states that:

> Patients with severe mechanical pain suggestive of spinal instability or any neurological signs or symptoms suggestive of MSCC should be nursed flat with neutral spine alignment, including log rolling or turning beds with use of a slipper pan for toilet until bony and neurological stability are ensured and cautious remobilisation may begin.

The Christie Trust in their guidelines for assessment of spinal stability propose that you:

> Assume the patient has spinal instability until investigations (MRI) prove otherwise.

They go on to say:

> The spine should be assumed to be 'unstable' until the Multi-Disciplinary Team decision agrees otherwise. NB: This decision should be made in the patient's local hospital.

This has important implications; the full baseline neurological assessment may need to take place whilst the patient is on flat bed rest. This could mean that the examination needs to be adapted considerably in a GP or physiotherapy clinic in a community setting. If a suspicion that suggests the cause of the symptoms is MSCC emerges during the consultation, consider if the patient needs to lay flat for the remainder of the examination. A local decision on these types of pathway is usually made and this will have implications for physiotherapy practice; familiarity with your own local pathway is essential. The following is an example of the Manchester Cancer Centre stability pathway (Fig. 8.3):

The gold standard investigation to confirm MSCC is whole spinal MRI. The MRI of the whole spine should be carried out and reported within 24 hours (NICE, 2008). Patients waiting for spinal surgery may continue to be nursed on flat bed rest whilst waiting for the MRI depending on the instructions from the spinal surgeon. After discussion with the wider MDT, a decision may be made for patients receiving radiotherapy to start careful mobilisation led by a specialist physiotherapy team. A small number of patients will not be suitable for either surgery or radiotherapy; these patients will have best supportive care and no treatment intervention. MDT agreement on careful mobilisation will instigate this approach. However, as with any Red Flag situation, continuous re-evaluation of the stability status is essential. Stabilisation with brace or collar may be considered, especially if severe pain is suffered and the patient is not suitable for surgery.

Intervention

Definitive treatment options are surgery, radiotherapy or symptom control. Those with no motor function for more than 48 hours are not likely to recover useful function after treatment. For those patients suffering significant pain, a single fraction of radiotherapy is often considered. It is important to remember that the goals of treatment for spinal metastases differ from the goals for primary tumour

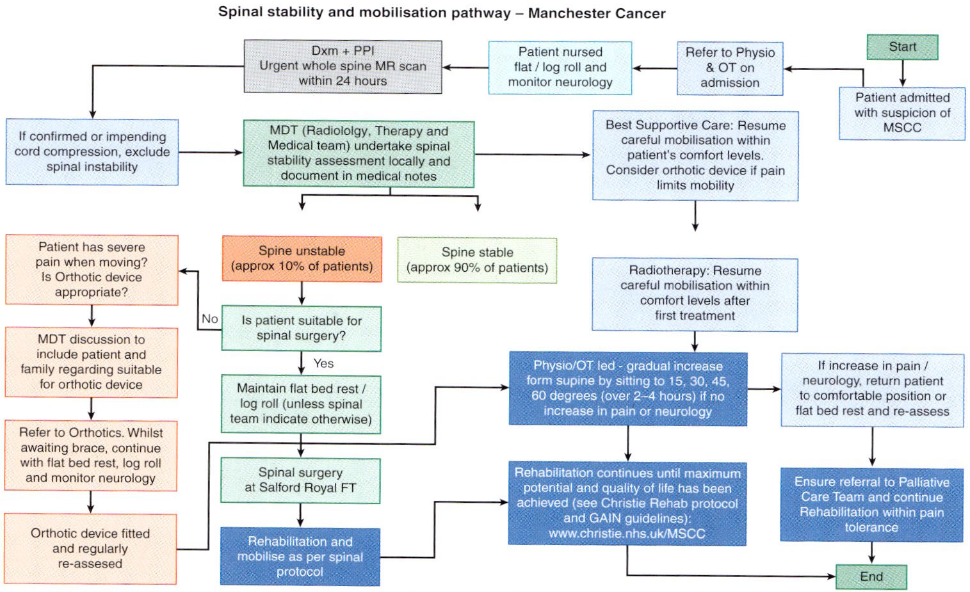

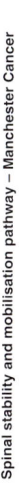

Spinal stability and mobilisation pathway – Manchester Cancer

Start

Patient admitted with suspicion of MSCC

Refer to Physio & OT on admission

Patient nursed flat / log roll and monitor neurology

Dxm + PPI
Urgent whole spine MR scan within 24 hours

If confirmed or impending cord compression, exclude spinal instability

MDT (Radiology, Therapy and Medical team) undertake spinal stability assessment locally and document in medical notes

Best Supportive Care: Resume careful mobilisation within patient's comfort levels. Consider orthotic device if pain limits mobility

Spine stable (approx 90% of patients)

Spine unstable (approx 10% of patients)

Is patient suitable for spinal surgery?

Yes

Maintain flat bed rest / log roll (unless spinal team indicate otherwise)

Spinal surgery at Salford Royal FT

Rehabilitation and mobilise as per spinal protocol

No

Patient has severe pain when moving? Is Orthotic device appropriate?

MDT discussion to include patient and family regarding suitable for orthotic device

Refer to Orthotics. Whilst awaiting brace, continue with flat bed rest, log roll and monitor neurology

Orthotic device fitted and regularly re-assessed

Radiotherapy: Resume careful mobilisation within comfort levels after first treatment

Physio/OT led - gradual increase form supine by sitting to 15, 30, 45, 60 degrees (over 2–4 hours) if no increase in pain or neurology

If increase in pain / neurology, return patient to comfortable position or flat bed rest and re-assess

Rehabilitation continues until maximum potential and quality of life has been achieved (see Christie Rehab protocol and GAIN guidelines) www.christie.nhs.uk/MSCC

Ensure referral to Palliative Care Team and continue Rehabilitation within pain tolerance

End

Fig. 8.3 **Assessment of spinal stability.** *DXM*, Dextromethorphan; *FT*, Foundation Trust; *MDT*, multidisciplinary team; *MRI*, magnetic resonance imaging; *MSCC*, metastatic spinal cord compression; *OT*, occupational therapy; *PPI*, proton pump inhibitor.

treatment as treatment intervention for spinal metastases is rarely curative. If metastases have developed, the primary concern of surgeons is to improve the overall quality of life and improve or maintain personal independence. Ultimately, this is achieved by decreasing pain and maintaining or relieving neurological impairment and spinal stability (Franic et al., 2016). It is judicious practice to engage with a spinal surgical team as soon as MSCC has been confirmed to optimise outcome for those patients considered suitable for surgery (Franic et al., 2016). This liaison is one of the principal roles of the MSCC coordinator. Patients presenting with suspected MSCC are initially treated with intravenous (IV) or oral corticosteroids plus a proton pump inhibitor for gastric protection, such as omeprazole. This initial steroid is administered to reduce oedema, hence alleviating pressure, in an attempt to improve pain and neurological compromise; dexamethasone is the steroid generally used. At this point, consideration of a surgical intervention will take place. Radiotherapy in non-surgical patients is administered within 24 hours and will aim to reduce the tumour size (Kaplow & Iyere, 2016). More detailed descriptions of each of the surgical and non-surgical modalities available for MSCC are beyond the scope of this book, but readers need to be aware that a multitude of treatment approaches are available. Combinations of approaches (such as radiotherapy and surgery) may be tried depending on the precise nature of the malignancy and performance status. An integrated MDT consisting of spinal surgeons, radiologists and oncologists is required to overcome the diagnostic and therapeutic challenges this complex patient group brings. Where available, the coordination of the communication and care by an MSCC coordinator cannot be underestimated when optimising patient outcome (NICE, 2008).

Surgery

Patchell et al. (2005) paved the way for surgical intervention and revolutionised practice. This treatment approach was later supported by Fehlings et al. (2016). The outcome is that patients who are fit enough for surgery are now more commonly offered surgical treatment for MSCC. Surgery could involve excision of the entire tumour or segment of it (Kaplow & Iyere, 2016). The increased incidence of surgical intervention is probably due to better clinical evidence, more robust surgical techniques and growing numbers of cancer sufferers (Morgen et al., 2013). Quraishi et al. (2013) suggest surgery should take place at the earliest possible convenience to optimise outcome. Their study identified that those undergoing surgery within 48 hours had better neurological outcome but that survival rates were not influenced.

For relatively fit patients with a good prognosis, decompressive surgery followed by radiotherapy is the recommended treatment approach. Identifying patients suitable for surgery early is a key milestone in maximising optimum prognosis and outcome. Radiotherapy can increase risk of wound breakdown and increase risk of infection threefold if taking place before surgery. Surgery may also aid diagnosis by obtaining a biopsy or enable stabilisation of any identified instability issues including pain. Major surgery is often only considered in those with a life expectancy of more than 3 months.

Favourable prognostic indicators for surgery are:
- histological findings (breast, prostate, renal, multiple myeloma, lymphoma)
- good ambulatory status at presentation
- good performance status

- a low number of comorbidities
- limited level spinal disease
- lack of visceral metastasis
- long interval between initial diagnosis and MSCC

For suitable surgical plus postoperative radiotherapy patients, the outcome for mobility, functional status, continence and pain control is more favourable compared with those undergoing radiotherapy alone. Early surgery may be more effective than radiotherapy at maintaining mobility in a subgroup of patients (Patchell et al., 2005; Nice, 2008). A life expectancy of 3–6 months is a much-quoted minimum requirement for major surgery to be considered (Miljenko et al., 2016). Wanman et al. (2017) point out that postoperative survival with MSCC depends on the type of primary tumour. However, surgery may maintain and improve ambulatory function. Surgical treatment is not always feasible and comes with significant risk. Palliative surgical procedures can be considered in some cases. Kyphoplasty and vertebroplasty, for example, may be considered appropriate for patients with shorter life expectancy if outcome and improved quality of life outweigh risk (Franic et al., 2016).

The goals of surgical treatment include stabilisation and pain control and preservation or improvement of function, including sphincter control, to enhance quality of life. Franic et al. (2016) list the goals of surgery as the following:

- control of tumour size
- pain reduction
- motor function preservation
- maintenance of sphincter control
- prevention of deformity
- upgrade and maintain quality of life remaining

Wanman et al. (2017) evaluated survival in 69 MSCC patients who underwent surgery. These patients had no history of cancer but presented with pain and/or neurological symptoms. Patients with cancer of unknown primary (CUP) had the shortest survival time at 3.5 months, myeloma and prostate cancer patients had the longest survival at 5 years and 6 years respectively. They concluded that postoperative survival for MSCC sufferers is strongly influenced by the type of primary tumour.

Radiotherapy

Unfortunately, the majority of patients presenting with MSCC will be unsuitable for surgery. Those unsuitable for surgery should receive radiotherapy within 24 hours of MRI diagnosis of MSCC. Radiotherapy at this stage is very effective in providing effective pain relief and aims to prevent further deterioration of the neurological status and potentially improve neurological function. Poorest survival is seen in those with a rapidly deteriorating picture with poor mobility, functional status and visceral involvement.

Rehabilitation

Most MSCC patients have extensive rehabilitation requirements, both as inpatients and as outpatients in the community. Thromboprophylaxis with compression stockings and low molecular weight heparin (if not surgical) is needed until mobile in an inpatient setting. Pressure area care until mobile is essential; mobilisation should ideally begin within 48 hours. Rehabilitation planning should begin from admission with onward liaison along local pathways into community-based healthcare, social services and hospices settings (Robson, 2014).

Although each individual modality may improve patients' symptoms, their combination provides the best outcome (Sodji et al., 2017). Pain is often further managed with a combination of analgesics and non-steroidal anti-inflammatory drugs; adjuvant therapies such as anticonvulsants or antidepressants may also be added to alleviate neuropathic pain (Kaplow & Iyere, 2016). Bisphosphonates are used to control metastatic bone symptoms, such as bone pain and pathological fractures, to strengthen the bones and guard against further fracture (Kaplow & Iyere, 2016).

Scoring systems to guide clinical decision-making

According to Franic et al. (2016), the decision-making process relating to onward management is assisted by the assimilation of a number of classification scoring systems and treatment algorithms, but clinical reasoning is essentially based on:

- primary tumour histology
- severity of impairment
- overall well-being
- likely benefit from surgery

Franic et al. (2016) go on to argue that it is reasonable to combine a number of systems to facilitate the clinical decision-making process. In essence, the information that forms the basis of clinical triage includes:

- extent of the disease, both vertebral and systemic
- degree of disability since the onset of new signs and symptoms
- duration of symptoms
- performance status prior to presentation and current state
- further lines of treatment available
- Tokuhashi score (Table 8.4)

TABLE 8.4 Tokuhashi revised prognostic scoring system for spinal metastasis.

	Score
1. General condition (Karnofsky Score)	
Poor (10%–40%)	0
Moderate (50%–70%)	1
Good (80%–100%)	2
2. Number of extra-spinal bone metastases	
≥3	0
1–2	1
0	2
3. Number of metastases in the vertebral body	
≥3	0
2	1
1	2
4. Metastases to major internal organs	
Unremovable	0
Removable	1
No metastases	2
5. Primary site of cancer	
Lung, osteosarcoma, stomach, bladder, oesophagus, pancreas	0
	1
Liver, gallbladder, unidentified	2
Others	3
Kidney, uterus	4
Rectum	5
Thyroid, breast, prostate, carcinoid tumour	
6. Palsy	
Complete (Frankel A, B)	0
Incomplete (Frankel C, D)	1
None (Frankel E)	2

Reproduced from Tokuhashi, Y., et al. A revised scoring system for preoperative evaluation of metastatic spine tumour prognosis. Spine. 2005;30(19):2186–2191.

The revised Tokuhashi scoring system is one of the more common scoring systems and is often used alongside other features for treatment guidance.

The cumulative Tokuhashi score of each of these variables suggests a predicted life expectancy.

Patients with a score of:

- 0–8 (predicted survival <6 months): conservative treatment
- 9–11 (predicted survival ≥6 months): palliative surgery or, rarely, excisional surgery for patients with a single lesion and no metastases to internal organs
- 12–15 (predicted survival of ≥1 year): excisional surgery

The clear message underpinning this chapter is that enhanced patient MSCC pathways promoting prompt diagnosis and treatment directly improve patient outcomes (Savage et al., 2014). A variety of authors agree that patients at risk of MSCC should be given information of what symptoms to be aware of to enable early diagnosis of MSCC (Hutchison et al., 2012). However, Savage et al. (2014), investigating perceptions of patients and staff, identified inconsistent findings. Fifty-six patients and 50 staff were involved in the study. A surprisingly low 4% of staff reported providing patients at risk of MSCC with information about the condition. Conversely, 20% of patients perceived that they had received information and 77% reported wanting that important information. This study identified that, in general, patients did not access additional information about MSCC once outside the healthcare setting. This underlines the importance of appropriate information being provided to those at risk of MSCC whilst undergoing healthcare to enable patients to be aware of MSCC and present in a timely manner if any suspicious symptoms develop (Hutchison et al., 2012). Notably, although spinal cord compression is most frequently seen in patients with adenocarcinomas such as breast, prostate, lung and renal cancer (Savage et al., 2014), any solid tumour could metastasise to the spine. Solid tumours that metastasise to the spine are known as adenocarcinomas (Hartvigsen et al., 2018). However, Frymoyer (1997) suggests 'don't ignore any history of cancer'; clinical decision-making will inform you of those at higher risk. It stands to reason that these patients should be safety netted in relation to the important Red Flags of MSCC of which to be aware. Unpublished Christie data identify that 27% of their patient population with no known bone metastasis develop MSCC. These cases are a challenge but neurology, function and quality of life can be preserved if patients receive rapid intervention (Bowers, 2015): working together we can make a difference! Just as in the case of cauda equina syndrome (CES) discussed earlier, patients at risk of MSCC need to be provided with clear information of what signs and symptoms to look out for and what to do should they occur (see previous chapter) to enhance early access to acute treatment (Hutchison et al., 2012).

Cases

The following are hypothetical cases to test your clinical decision-making.

Hilda is a 60-year-old woman with back pain and a previous history of breast cancer.

- Should you organise an MRI?
- Should it be whole spine?

You need to know more information and the subjective examination is key in clinically reasoning onward management. Consider the Red Flags mnemonic described earlier in Chapter 7 and presented on the credit card (Fig. 7.4) and NICE guidelines listed above. If none are currently present, do not forget the power of 'watchful wait' and see how things develop, carefully safety netting the patient by telling them of signs and symptoms to be aware of. If Red Flags do develop, then a whole spine MRI is the gold standard image of choice to exclude spinal metastases.

(A) Hilda tells you that her cancer was described as 'aggressive' at diagnosis. She had lymph node involvement. These were removed and her breast cancer was described as HER positive. Hilda appears disproportionately distressed about her back pain.
- What now?
- Consider whole spinal MRI within 7 days
- Safety netting

(B) You have no clinical notes for Hilda in your clinic. Hilda knows little of her breast cancer but she does know that she had her lymph nodes removed. Hilda has a 40-year history of back pain. The pain is in the same place that it has always been; however, the quality of the pain has changed and she now describes sudden severe episodes of pain, especially at night.
- What now?
- Whole spinal MRI within 7 days
- Safety net

(C) Hilda has severe pain disturbing sleep and is unable to lie flat during the examination. She is sleeping in a chair at night now due to the pain; her lower limbs are pain free, and bladder and bowel function are normal, although a little constipated with medication. However, Hilda is finding that her legs feel heavy and peculiar and she is tripping and stumbling.

She attributes this clumsiness to the severe pain. Neurological examination including sensation to light touch, pin prick and proprioception are all normal.

- What now?
- Consider your local MSCC pathway including whole spinal MRI within 24 hours. Does your pathway nurse the patient supine at the stage? If so you may be required to nurse flat immediately.

The Blue Light is on

Let us return to where this book began.

It is Friday afternoon and it is 4 pm

Your next patient is Barbara, a 62-year-old woman. She presents with an 18-month history of low back pain and bilateral leg symptoms. She has been referred to you by the local physiotherapy department. She was previously seen by a consultant neurologist 8 months earlier and a lumbar spine MRI was carried out. Degenerative changes only were identified with no neurological compromise. The neurologist referred Barbara on for physiotherapy. The problem with low back pain and bilateral leg pain has continued to progress very slowly, with a sudden deterioration over the last 2 months. Barbara complains of increasing hip pain, bilateral leg pain and paraesthesia in both legs. She complains of extra-segmental numbness in both legs, affecting both the anterior and posterior aspects of the legs to the ankles with pins and needles in both feet. The paraesthesia in the feet is intermittent and particularly worse in the morning. Barbara reports a recent onset of tripping and falling and feels as if she is losing all the feeling in both legs. She describes feeling unsteady with poor balance.

Over the last 4 weeks she describes hesitancy in relation to bladder control, with frequency of passing small amounts of urine. She can tell when she has finished passing urine and sensation when she wipes herself after toileting is normal. She describes pain first thing in the morning as 7/10 on a numeric pain rating scale but, as the day progresses, so does the pain, increasing to 10/10. Barbara said that in the previous 18 months she had lost 9 kg (20 lb) in weight but this unexplained weight loss has now stabilised. This weight loss equates to approximately 10% of her body weight over an 18-month period. To help attend this appointment, she needed morphine to control her symptoms. Sleep is very disturbed due to pain and she describes getting stuck in positions due to pain when she tries to roll over during the night.

On examination, the unsteadiness on her legs is obvious. She stands with a wide-based gait but demonstrates a fairly good range of movement. Objectively, there is no neurology to find, including reflexes, and abdominal palpation was negative. Current medication is morphine twice a day, ibuprofen three times a day, paracetamol three times a day and pregabalin three times a day.

Past medical history

Barbara has a history of cervical spinal fusion. She underwent an operation 11 years ago for a C6–7-disc protrusion with C7 root entrapment producing left arm pain and weakness. Complete recovery was achieved postoperatively.

She is a 10 per day smoker and has smoked for 40 years, drinks minimal amounts of alcohol and has no history of TB or cancer.

We left you with the following questions:

What are your diagnostic alternatives?

What investigations will you organise and when?

Your diagnostic alternatives include the following:

- MSCC
- CES
- Cord compression for a number of other reasons including
- Osteoporotic collapse, infection, disc lesion

At this point, further investigations of the spine are the only way of establishing the most likely diagnosis. (Of note: if the spinal examination is negative, investigations of the pelvic cavity must be considered.)

What investigations of the spine will you organise?

From the differential diagnosis perspective, the stability issue relating to MSCC has the heaviest clinical weighting; therefore, excluding MSCC first is the strongest driver for onward medical management (refer). Hence, the MSCC pathway, including whole spinal MRI within 24 hours, would be the suggested pathway in this case at this stage of Barbara's journey. NICE guidelines (2008) would suggest at this stage supine lying until spinal stability is assessed but local pathways are key to management at this stage.

However, Barbara's whole spinal MRI identified the following:

- Disc bulge at C4/5 impinging on the cord with resultant signal change
- A large central disc at L3/4 causing cauda equina compression

In addition, Barbara's blood test results, along with serum and urine electrophoresis, were carried out; these were entirely normal. Barbara was presenting with incomplete CES (CES-I) (Figure 5.7).

Action

- Urgent referral to spinal team

Outcome
- Barbara underwent emergency surgery and had an extremely positive outcome

This is what Barbara said after her surgery:

> It's only afterwards when you look up the symptoms and you see how close I came – it's almost what could have happened, I am just thankful that I got there in time and okay I might not be able to walk 20 odd miles a day any more but I can walk and to me that's the most important thing and as I said to you the first time. My priority is that I want to dance at my daughter's wedding and now I feel I can...

and she did dance at her daughter's wedding. A later interview identified that Barbara was delighted that she danced in '...killer heels'.

So, we come to the end of the last chapter but we would like to leave you with our final message: working with patients as partners, safety netting those at risk of serious conditions, remaining clinically vigilant at each patient consultation, keeping up to date with the latest evidence and knowing local pathways will ensure that we can and will continue to make a difference to patient care for those suffering from serious spinal pathology.

References

Bowers B. Recognising metastatic spinal cord compression. *Br J Community Nurs.* 2015;20(4):162–165.

Brooks F, Ghatahora A, Brooks M, et al. Management of metastatic spinal cord compression; awareness of NICE guidance. *Eur J Surg Traumatol.* 2014;1;S255–9.

Christie NHS FT web site. Immediate management of suspected MSCC. http://www.christie.nhs.uk.

Fehlings M, Nater A, Tetreault L, et al. Survival and clinical outcome in surgically treated patients with metastatic epidural spinal cord compression: results of a prospective multicentre AOspine study. *J Clin Oncol*. 2016;34(3):268–276.

Fisher CG, DiPaola CP, Ryken TC, et al. A novel classification system for spinal instability in neoplastic disease: an evidence-based approach and expert consensus from the Spine Oncology Study Group. *Spine (Phila Pa 1976)*. 2010;2010(35):E1221–E1229.

Fox S, Spiess M, Hnenny L, Fourney D. Spinal Instability neoplastic score (SINS); Reliability among spinal fellows and resident physicians in orthopaedic surgery and neurosurgery. *Global Spine J*. 2017;7(8):744–748.

Franic M, Bilic V, Dokuzovic S, et al. Surgical treatment of metastatic disease of the vertebral column. *Acta Clin Croat*. 2016;55(3):474–482.

Frymoyer JW. *The Adult Spine: Principles and Practice*. Lippincott-Raven Publishers; 1997.

Hartvigsen J, Hancock M, Kongsted A, et al. Low Back Pain 1: what low back pain is and why we need to pay attention. Lancet low Back Pain Series Working Group. *Lancet*. 2018;391:P2356–2367.

Hutchison C, Morrison A, Rice A, Tait G, Haeden S. Provision of information about malignant spinal cord compression: perception of patients and staff. *Int J Palliative Nurs*. 2012;18(2):61–68.

Kaplow R, Iyere K. Oncology emergency series. Understanding spinal cord compression. *Nursing 2016*. 2016;46(9):44–50.

Levack P, Collie D, Gibson A, et al. *A prospective Audit of the Diagnosis, Management and Outcome of Malignant Spinal Cord Compression CRAG 97/08*. Edinburgh: CRAG; 2001.

Miljenko F, Vide B, Stjepan D, Stjepan C, Tomislav C, Kresimir R. Surgical treatment of metastatic disease of the vertebral column. *Acta Clin Croat*. 2016;55:474–482.

Morgen S, Lund-Andersen C, Larsen C, Engelholm S, Dahl B. Prognosis in patients with metastatic spinal cord compression: survival in different cancer diagnosis in a cohort of 2321 patients. *Spine (Phila Pa 1976)*. 2013;38(16):1362–1367.

NICE (2008) Clinical guideline [CG75] Published date: November 2008. https://www.nice.org.uk/Guidance/CG75.

Patchell R, Tibbs P, Regine W, et al. Direct decompressive surgical resection in the treatment of spinal cord compression caused by metastatic cancer: a randomised trial. *Lancet*. 2005;366:643–648.

Pease N, Harris r Finlay I. Development and audit of a care pathway for the management of patients with suspected malignant spinal cord compression. *Physiotherapy*. 2004;90:27–34.

Quraishi NA, Rajagopal T, Manoharan S, Elsayed S, Edwards K, Boszczyk B. Effect of timing of surgery on neurological outcome and survival in metastatic spinal cord compression. *Eur Spine*. 2013;6:1383–1388.

Richards L, Misra V, Greenhalgh S. *The Manchester and Cheshire MSCC Service* (poster). 2016.

Robson P. Metastatic Spinal Cord Compression; a rare but important complication of cancer. *Clin Med (Lond)*. 2014;14(5):542–545.

Savage P, Sharkey R, Kua T, et al. Malignant spinal cord compression: NICE guidance, improvements and challenges. *QJM*. 2014;(4):277–282.

Sodji Q, Kaminski J, Willey C, Kim N, Mourad W, Vender J, Dasher B. Management of metastatic spinal cord compression. *South Med J*. 2017;110(9):586–593.

Wanman J, Grabowski P, Nystrom H, et al. Metastatic spinal cord compression as the first sign of malignancy. *Acta Orthop*. 2017;88(4):457–462.

White N. Metastatic spinal cord compression, presentation, diagnosis and management. *Hospital Medicine Clinics*. 2016;5(3):452–465.

Index

Note: Page numbers followed by "f" indicate figures "t" indicate tables and "b" indicate boxes.